Small Animal Bandaging, Casting, and Splinting Techniques

Small Animal Bandaging, Casting, and Splinting Techniques

Steven F. Swaim, DVM, MS
Professor Emeritus
Scott-Ritchey Research Center *and*
Dept. of Clinical Sciences
College of Veterinary Medicine
Auburn University, Alabama

Walter C. Renberg, DVM, MS, Dip. ACVS
Associate Professor
Department of Clinical Sciences
College of Veterinary Medicine
Kansas State University
Manhattan, Kansas

Kathy M. Shike, RVT
Veterinary Technician
Department of Clinical Sciences
College of Veterinary Medicine
Kansas State University
Manhattan, Kansas

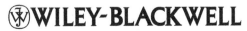
A John Wiley & Sons, Inc., Publication

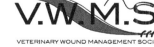
VETERINARY WOUND MANAGEMENT SOCIETY

Edition first published 2011

© 2011 Steven F. Swaim, Walter C. Renberg, and Kathy M. Shike

Blackwell Publishing was acquired by John Wiley & Sons in February 2007. Blackwell's publishing program has been merged with Wiley's global Scientific, Technical, and Medical business to form Wiley-Blackwell.

Editorial Office
2121 State Avenue, Ames, Iowa 50014-8300, USA

For details of our global editorial offices, for customer services, and for information about how to apply for permission to reuse the copyright material in this book, please see our Website at www.wiley.com/wiley-blackwell.

Authorization to photocopy items for internal or personal use, or the internal or personal use of specific clients, is granted by Blackwell Publishing, provided that the base fee is paid directly to the Copyright Clearance Center, 222 Rosewood Drive, Danvers, MA 01923. For those organizations that have been granted a photocopy license by CCC, a separate system of payments has been arranged. The fee code for users of the Transactional Reporting Service is ISBN-13: 978-0-8138-1962-4/2011.

Wiley also publishes its books in a variety of electronic formats. Some content that appears in print may not be available in electronic books.

Designations used by companies to distinguish their products are often claimed as trademarks. All brand names and product names used in this book are trade names, service marks, trademarks, or registered trademarks of their respective owners. The publisher is not associated with any product or vendor mentioned in this book. This publication is designed to provide accurate and authoritative information in regard to the subject matter covered. It is sold on the understanding that the publisher is not engaged in rendering professional services. If professional advice or other expert assistance is required, the services of a competent professional should be sought.

Library of Congress Cataloging-in-Publication Data

Swaim, Steven F.
  Small animal bandaging, casting, and splinting techniques / Steven F. Swaim, Walter C. Renberg, and Kathy M. Shike.
     p. ; cm.
  Includes bibliographical references and index.
  ISBN 978-0-8138-1962-4 (pbk. : alk. paper)
  1. Pet medicine.   2. Veterinary surgical emergencies.   3. Bandages and bandaging.   4. Surgical casts.   5. Splints (Surgery) I. Renberg, Walter C.   II. Shike, Kathy M.   III. Title.
  [DNLM: 1. Bandages--veterinary.   2. Orthopedic Fixation Devices--veterinary.   3. Animals, Domestic.   4. Wounds and Injuries--veterinary. SF 914.3]
  SF914.3.S93 2011
  636.089'71--dc22
                          2010042171

A catalog record for this book is available from the U.S. Library of Congress.

Set in 9.5 on 11.5 pt Palatino by Toppan Best-set Premedia Limited
Printed in ••

Disclaimer
The publisher and the authors make no representations or warranties with respect to the accuracy or completeness of the contents of this work and specifically disclaim all warranties, including without limitation warranties of fitness for a particular purpose. No warranty may be created or extended by sales or promotional materials. The advice and strategies contained herein may not be suitable for every situation. This work is sold with the understanding that the publisher is not engaged in rendering legal, accounting, or other professional services. If professional assistance is required, the services of a competent professional person should be sought. Neither the publisher nor the author shall be liable for damages arising herefrom. The fact that an organization or Website is referred to in this work as a citation and/or a potential source of further information does not mean that the authors or the publisher endorses the information the organization or Website may provide or recommendations it may make. Further, readers should be aware that Internet Websites listed in this work may have changed or disappeared between when this work was written and when it is read.

1   2011

Dedication

This book is dedicated to the veterinarians, veterinary technicians, residents, interns, veterinary students, and especially the animals that will benefit from its use.

Table of Contents

Veterinary Wound Management Society Mission

"The mission of the Veterinary Wound Management Society is to advance the art and science of animal wound management, thus promoting excellence in the field."

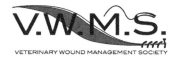

Foreword

Bandage application is a daily activity in most small animal practices. Challenges arise due to variations in size, shape, injury type and location, activity level, and desire (or lack thereof!) to keep a bandage in place posed by our veterinary patients. Successful bandaging is both an art and a science. *The art:* thinking outside the box for creative solutions to protect injuries in even the most awkward of locations. *The science:* selecting bandage components that work positively with the biology of wound healing and use the laws of physics to advantage. This book successfully incorporates both.

As so aptly stated in chapter I, sound clinical judgment is important when applying and modifying bandages. The authors of this book have a wealth of expertise in managing wounds in veterinary patients and are major contributors to the research that backs up these techniques. Indeed, Dr. Steven F. Swaim's name is synonymous with wound management in veterinary medicine; veterinary patients worldwide are the beneficiaries of his extensive scholarship in the field and his passion for teaching with which he so successfully educates members of the veterinary profession. Dr. Walter C. Renberg is a veterinary surgeon and teacher with wide-ranging clinical and research experience who brings his specialized knowledge of orthopedic injury and biomechanics to the subject of bandaging. Ms. Kathy M. Shike has extensive hands-on bandaging experience as a small animal surgery technician and instructor for veterinary students and has contributed to many research projects in the field. The clinical and research experiences of the authors are translated here into a format that the reader can use to make sound bandaging decisions for his or her own patients.

Step-by-step illustrated instructions on a range of bandaging techniques are a unique component of this book and provide a very practical, visual guide. Specific instructions on bandage application are rounded out by clearly organized information on the indications, aftercare, safe removal or modification, and potential complications of each bandage type. This material is further enhanced by plenty of helpful tips stemming from the extensive personal experiences of the authors. Throughout the text there is an emphasis on patient comfort and selecting a bandage type that will best support healing in each individual.

As current president of the Veterinary Wound Management Society, I would like to say that the VWMS is exceptionally pleased to endorse *Small Animal Bandaging, Casting, and Splinting Techniques*. The authors have expertly integrated the art and science of bandaging into a very clinically applicable text. This book will be a frequently used and most welcome resource for practitioners and trainees alike in the veterinary profession.

Bonnie Grambow Campbell, DVM, PhD,
Diplomate ACVS
Veterinary Wound Management Society, President
Clinical Assistant Professor of Small Animal
Surgery, Washington State University

Preface

Veterinarians are often presented with animals that have wounds of varying severity and orthopedic injuries of a like nature. A major part of the therapy of these conditions is the bandaging, casting, and splinting necessary in their treatment. To be effective, these applications must be properly constructed, securely held in place, and protected from molestation. The purpose of this book is to describe in text and pictures techniques that the authors have found effective in applying these structures. In addition, for each bandage, cast, or splint, the indications, aftercare, and advantages and complications are presented.

Acknowledgments

We acknowledge the work of Dave Adams and Chris Barker for their photographic contribution to the book. The word processing skills of Mrs. Barbara Webster are appreciated, and gratitude goes to Brooke Grieger for the artwork in the book.

Small Animal Bandaging, Casting, and Splinting Techniques

1 Basics of Bandaging, Casting, and Splinting

Bandaging

Purposes and functions of a bandage

Bandages serve many functions in wound management (table 1.1). In general, bandages provide an environment that promotes wound healing.

Table 1.1. Properties of a bandage.

- Provide an aesthetic appearance
- Wound protection from environmental contamination
- Prevention of interference from the patient
- Prevention of tissue damage by desiccation
- Provide a moist environment to promote healing
- Retain heat and create an acid environment for oxygen dissociation to tissue
- Provide pain relief
- Immobilization of wound edges
- Provide pressure to close dead space and reduce edema and hemorrhage
- Deliver topical medications
- Absorb exudate
- Debride wounds
- Help stabilize concurrent orthopedic injuries

Sources: Williams, John, and Moores, Allison. 2009. *BSAVA Manual of Canine and Feline Wound Management and Reconstruction*, 2nd ed., pp. 37–53. Quedgeley, Gloucester, England: British Small Animal Veterinary Association.

Hedlund, Cheryl S. 2007. Surgery of the integumentary system. In *Small Animal Surgery*, 3rd ed., pp. 159–259. St. Louis, MO: Mosby, Elsevier.

Samll Animal Bandaging, Casting, and Splinting Techniques   Steven F. Swaim, Walter C. Renberg, and Kathy M. Shike
© Steven F. Swaim, Walter C. Renberg, and Kathy M. Shike

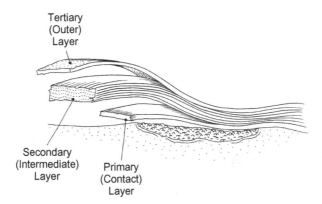

Fig. 1.1.   The three layers of a bandage: primary-contact layer, secondary-intermediate layer, and tertiary-outer layer.

Components of a bandage

There are three components or layers of a bandage. These are the primary, secondary, and tertiary bandage layers (fig. 1.1).

Primary-contact layer

The primary layer is also called the contact layer. It is directly in contact with the wound. Depending on the stage of healing, this layer can be used to debride tissue, absorb exudates, deliver medication, or form an occlusive seal over the wound. The primary layer plays a vital role in providing a wound environment that promotes healing rather than a layer that just covers the wound. The properties of primary dressing materials vary widely, and it is important to select a primary dressing that is appropriate to the wound in its current stage of healing and to change the type of dressing as healing progresses. Occlusiveness and absorption are important properties of the contact dressing.

Highly absorptive dressings
Highly absorptive dressings are indicated in the treatment of wounds that are heavily contaminated or infected, have foreign debris present, and/or are producing large amounts of exudate. Such wounds are generally in the early inflammatory stage of wound healing. Once a wound has entered the later inflammatory or early repair stage, another form of dressing is selected that will promote the progression of the healing process, for example, a moisture-retentive dressing.

Gauze dressings   Gauge dressings are used in wet-to-dry and dry-to-dry bandages. These forms of bandage are older techniques for bandaging and provide a means of clearing a wound of exudates and necrotic tissue in the early days of wound management. For instance, dry gauze may be the most economical primary dressing in a highly productive wound where absorptive bandage changes are needed multiple times daily. However, after three to five days, a contact layer that will promote wound repair is indicated, for example, calcium alginate, hydrogel, or foam dressing.

With wet-to-dry dressings wide mesh gauze is wetted with sterile saline, lactated Ringers solution, or 0.05% chlorhexidine diacetate solution and is placed in wounds with viscous exudate or necrotic tissue. The exudates are diluted and absorbed into the secondary bandage layer. As the fluid evaporates, the bandage dries and adheres to the wound. When the dressing is removed, adhered necrotic tissue is also removed. Removal is usually painful. Thus, moistening the gauze with warm 2% lidocaine that does not contain epinephrine makes removal more comfortable. In cats, moistening the gauze with warm physiologic saline is indicated.

For dry-to-dry dressings, dry gauze is placed in a wound that has low-viscosity exudate. The exudate is absorbed and evaporates from the bandage, leaving the dressing adhered to the wound. Removal of the dressing removes necrotic tissue. Moistening the gauze with warm 2% lidocaine makes removal more comfortable. Moistening the gauze with warm physiologic saline should be done in cats.

These gauze dressings have several disadvantages: (1) Both healthy and unhealthy tissue are removed at dressing change. (2) The dry environment does not favor the function of cells and proteases involved in healing. (3) There is danger of exogenous bacteria wicking inward toward the wound with a wet gauze, and if the dressing is maintained wet tissue maceration can occur. (4) Dry gauze can disperse bacteria into the air at bandage change. (5) Fibers of the gauze can remain adhered to the wound to induce inflammation. (6) The adherent dressings are more painful to wear and to remove. (7) Removal of wound fluid with the dressings removes cytokines and growth factors essential for optimal healing.

Hypertonic saline dressings   These dressings are a good choice for infected or necrotic, heavily exudative wounds that need aggressive debridement. Their 20% sodium chloride content gives them an osmotic effect to draw fluid from the wound to decrease edema and thus enhance circulation. The osmotic action also desiccates tissue and bacteria. These dressings are changed every one to two days until necrosis and infection are under control. The debridement of this osmotic dressing is nonselective in that both healthy and necrotic tissue are removed at dressing change. The dressings are used early in wound treatment to convert a necrotic sloughing wound to a moderately exudating granulating wound. At this time the primary dressing is changed to a calcium alginate, hydrogel, or foam dressing.

Calcium alginate dressings   These hydrophilic dressings are indicated in moderate to highly exudative wounds, that is, wounds in the inflammatory stage of healing. However, their placement over exposed bone, muscle, tendon, and dry necrotic tissue is not recommended. Neither should they be used on dry wounds or those covered by dry necrotic tissue. They are available as a feltlike material in pad or rope form. The calcium alginate, which is derived from seaweed, interacts with sodium in wound fluids to create a sodium alginate gel that maintains a moist wound environment.

Attention should be paid to the hydration of wound tissues when using calcium alginate dressings. To help maintain a moist environment, the dressing can be overlaid with a vapor-permeable polyurethane sheet. However, if too much exudate is being produced in the presence of the dressing, it can be covered with an absorptive foam dressing. Because it is so absorptive, it can dehydrate a wound as the healing progresses and exudate decreases. If it is left in a wound too long, it dehydrates and hardens to form a calcium alginate eschar that is difficult to remove. Rehydrating it back to a gel with saline aids in its removal.

These dressings aid in the transition from the inflammatory to the repair phase of healing by promoting autolytic debridement and granulation tissue formation. The dressing can be premoistened with saline to promote granulation tissue in wounds without considerable exudate. Additional benefits of this dressing include a hemostatic property and entrapment of bacteria in the gel that can be lavaged from the wound at dressing change.

Copolymer starch dressings   This type of highly absorptive dressing is indicated for necrotic infected wounds that are moderately to highly exudative. If an occlusive cover is needed to hold them in place or retain some moisture, they can be overlaid with a hydrocolloid dressing. At dressing change, the polymer is removed by lavage.

It is important to observe the exudate level in wounds being treated with copolymer starch dressings. If exudate levels become too low, the dressing adheres to the wound. This can result in tissue damage when it is removed and inflammation if fragments of dressing are left in the wound.

Moisture-retentive dressings

Moisture-retentive dressings (MRDs) provide a warm, moist environment over a wound in which cell proliferation and function are enhanced in the inflammatory and repair stages of healing. In addition,

Table 1.2. Advantages of moisture-retentive dressings (MRDs)*.

- Barrier against exogenous bacteria
- Prevent tissue desiccation
- Improved concentration of systemically administered antibiotics
- White blood cells stay in the wound with their enzymatic activity for autolytic debridement
- Low oxygen tension to lower pH and deter bacterial growth, favor collagen synthesis, enhance angiogenesis, and attract white blood cells
- Maintain physiologic temperature to support cell function, proteases, and growth factors
- Comfort when in place and when removed
- Waterproof against urine and other fluids
- Decreased bandage changes and cost
- Decreased scarring
- Less aerosolization of bacteria at bandage change

Source: Campbell, Bonnie Grambow. 2006. Dressings, bandages, and splints for wound management in dogs and cats. *Veterinary Clinics of North America: Small Animal Practice.* 36(4):759–91. Philadelphia: Saunders/Elsevier.

*MRDs will vary in their possession of these advantages.

the retained fluid provides a physiologic ratio of proteases, protease inhibitors, growth factors, and cytokines at each stage of healing. Thus, exudate can be beneficial in healing. Clinical judgment should be used in deciding whether treatment should begin with one of the highly absorbent dressings first and then change to an MRD or whether treatment can begin with an MRD. In general, a highly absorptive dressing should be considered initially if there is a great amount of necrosis, foreign debris, infection, and exudate.

The wound environment under an MRD provides several advantages in the progression of wound healing (table 1.2). There are disadvantages of MRDs in that retained fluid can cause maceration (softening caused by trapped moisture) and excoriation (damage caused by excess proteolytic enzymes) of the periwound skin.

Polyurethane foam dressings   The dressings are soft, compressible, nonadherent, highly conforming dressings. They are highly absorptive by wicking action and are designed for use in moderate to highly exudative wounds. The foam dressings maintain a moist environment and support autolytic debridement. In addition, they can promote the formation of healthy granulation tissue and have been reported to promote epithelialization. Thus, they are a dressing that can be used in both the inflammatory and the repair stages of healing. An alternative way to use the foam is to saturate it with liquid medication for delivery to the wound.

The frequency of bandage change with foams is related to the stage of wound healing. It can vary from one to seven days, with the shorter times between changes being in the early stages of management when there is considerable fluid production.

Polyurethane film dressings   These film dressings are thin, transparent, flexible, semiocclusive (permeable to gas but not water or bacteria) sheets. They have an adhesive perimeter for attaching them to periwound skin, and their transparency allows wound visualization. They are nonabsorptive and should be used on wounds with no or minimal exudate. For instance, they are suited for dry necrotic eschars, or shallow wounds, such as partial-thickness wounds like abrasions. They can also be used on wounds in the advanced repair stage of healing where there is need for a moist environment to promote epithelialization. Another use of the films is as a cover over other contact layers to support moisture retention and to provide a bacteria and waterproof cover.

The films should not be used on wounds that have high levels of exudate, are infected, or have fragile periwound skin. Neither should they be used on wounds over exposed bone, muscle, or tendon or on deep burns.

The dressings do not adhere well to areas with skin folds or unshaved hair. Hair growth on the periwound skin can push the adhesive attachment of the dressing off of the skin. However, adherence can be improved around the perimeter of the wound with vapor-permeable film spray.

With this type of dressing, the cloudy white to yellow exudate that accumulates under the dressing should not be interpreted as infection. It is just wound surface exudate. Infection will present as heat, swelling, pain, and hyperemia of the surrounding tissues.

Hydrogel dressings   Hydrogels are water-rich gel dressings that are in the form of a sheet or an amorphorus hydrogel. Some hydrogels contain other medications that can be beneficial to wound healing, such as acemannan, a wound healing stimulant, and metronidazole or silver sulfadiazine, antimicrobials.

Because they donate moisture to a wound, the hydrogels can be used in wounds with an eschar or dry sloughing tissue to rehydrate the tissues. To assure that wound moisture is transferred to the tissue and not the secondary bandage layer, the hydrogel can be overlaid with a nonadherent semiocclusive dressing or vapor-permeable polyurethane foam. Some hydrogels have an impermeable covering as part of the dressing. Conversely to donating fluid to wounds, some hydrogels are able to absorb considerable fluid and can be used in exudative wounds. These dressings can also be used in necrotic wounds to provide a moist environment to promote autolytic debridement and aid in granulation tissue formation.

In noninfected full-thickness wounds, the dressings are generally changed every three days. However, if a hydrogel containing a wound healing stimulant or antimicrobial is being used, daily change may be indicated to maintain their activity in the wound. With abrasions that have minimal exudate, hydrogels may be changed every four to seven days. At dressing change, the hydrogel is removed from the wound with gentle saline irrigation.

Hydrocolloid dressings   Hydrocolloid dressings are a combination of absorbent and elastomeric components that interact with wound fluid to form a gel. Some dressings have an adhesive layer of hydrocolloid that contacts the wound and a outer occlusive polyurethane film. The hydrocolloid adheres to the periwound skin, and the dressing over the wound interacts with wound fluid to produce an occlusive gel. The gel may have a mild odor and yellow purulent appearance. However, this should not be interpreted as infection. Infection of the wound will be manifested by heat, swelling, pain, and hyperemia of the wound and periwound tissues. The gel is usually more tenacious than just exudate or the gel associated with hydrogel dressings.

Although the dressings are available in a paste as well as granular and powdered form, they are generally used as the sheet form that provides a thermally insulated moist environment which is impermeable to fluid, gas, and bacteria.

Hydrocolloids can be used in partial or full-thickness wounds with clean or necrotic bases, including pressure wounds, minor burns, abrasions, or graft donor sites. They can be used in both the inflammatory and repair stages of healing. In the inflammatory stage of healing they promote autolytic debridement. In the repair stage of healing they stimulate granulation tissue, collagen synthesis, and epithelialization. However, their adherence to periwound skin may delay wound contraction. The dressings should not be used in heavily infected wounds or wounds producing large amounts of exudate. The large amounts of exudate can lead to maceration and excoriation of periwound skin.

For application, the skin around the wound should be clipped. The pad is warmed between the hands and cut to be about 2 cm larger than the wound. After removing the backing, it is placed over the wound. The tacky nature of the dressing allows it to stick to the periwound skin. At about two to three days, the dressing should be changed when it feels like a fluid-filled blister over the wound and before the underlying gel leaks from around the edges. After removal of the dressing, the gel is lavaged or gently wiped from the wound and periwound skin, respectively. Use of the dressing should be discontinued when the wound is fully epithelialized.

Nonadherent semiocclusive dressings   These dressings have a low absorptive capacity. They are porous and allow fluid to move through them into the secondary bandage layer where it can evaporate. This porosity could also allow exogenous bacteria to penetrate toward the wound.

These dressings can be either a wide mesh gauze impregnated with petrolatum or an absorbent material encased in a perforated nonadherent material. Although they are classified as nonadherent, they are actually low adherent. With the petrolatum-impregnated gauze, the granulation tissue or epithelium can grow into the meshes and thus adhere to the wound, resulting in tissue damage when they are removed. With the perforated nonadherent material, the pad can adhere to the wound when the wound dries and exudate dries in the perforations. Granulation tissue and epithelium can also enter the perforations if they are large enough.

If the petrolatum-impregnated gauze is used in the repair stage of healing, it should be used in the early repair stage, and it should be changed often enough so the granulation tissue does not grow into the meshes. Because petrolatum may interfere with epithelialization, its early use will prevent its interference with epithelialization. Once epithelialization starts, the perforated nonadherent material with absorbent filler should be used.

If the perforated nonadherent material with absorbent filler is used, its purpose is to retain some moisture over the wound to promote epithelialization and allow excess fluid to be absorbed into the secondary layer. It should be used on superficial wounds with low to moderate levels of exudate. They are often used in the latter part of the repair stage when exudate levels are low. They are also a good primary layer for sutured wounds.

Antimicrobial dressings

Antimicrobial agents such as iodine, silver, polyhexamethylene biguanide, activated charcoal, and antibiotics have been incorporated into dressings. These dressings are indicated to treat infected wounds or wounds at risk for infection. The dressings are not moisture retentive. Thus, covering them with a polyurethane film dressing may keep them from drying out.

Dressings containing cadexomer iodine release iodine into the wound without having a negative effect on wound cells. The slow release of iodine is designed to maintain adequate levels of active iodine for about 48 hours.

Silver ions in dressings have a broad antimicrobial effect and can be effective against otherwise antibiotic-resistant organisms to include some mycotic organisms. Such dressings are available in various forms to include gauze, gauze roll, low adherent, hydrocolloid, hydrogel, and alginate dressings.

Polyhexamethylene biguanide (PHMB) is an antiseptic related to chlorhexidine. It has been incorporated in gauze sponges and roll gauze to provide an antimicrobial dressing. It is bactericidal, and bacteria do not develop a resistance to this broad-spectrum compound. It is tissue compatible and does not have any apparent effects on wound healing. The PHMB has a prolonged antibacterial effect; it prevents bacteria on the wound from contaminating the environment and stops exogenous bacteria from penetrating the bandage.

Activated charcoal dressings provide a moist wound environment. They also absorb bacteria, prevent exuberant granulation tissue formation, and reduce wound odor.

Gentamicin-impregnated collagen sponges of type I bovine collagen provide high levels of antibiotic at the site of placement, while serum levels remain below toxic levels. These dressings have also been reported to have a hemostatic effect.

Extracellular matrix bioscaffold dressings

Extracellular matrix dressings (ECMs) are acellular biodegradable sheets with a three-dimensional ultrastructure. They are derived from porcine small intestinal submucosa or porcine urinary bladder submucosa matrix. The dressings contain structural proteins, growth factors, cytokines, and their inhibitors. Over the first two weeks of its presence in a wound, there is degradation of the scaffold, with the degradation products being chemotactic for repair cells. The repair cells enter the wound as stem cells that deposit a site-specific matrix. In other words, if the dressing has been placed in a skin wound, the matrix will be like that of skin/dermis. By 30 to 90 days, the entire bioscaffold is replaced by site-specific tissue.

ECMs are unique in the way they are applied. The wound must be thoroughly debrided and free of topical medications, cleaning agents, and exudates. Infection should be eliminated or well controlled. The sheet is cut to a size slightly larger than the wound, rehydrated with saline, tucked beneath the skin at the wound edge, and sutured in place. If drainage is expected, it can be fenestrated. A nonadhesive or moisture-retentive dressing is placed over the ECM. At the first bandage change in three to four days, all parts of the bandage are changed except the ECM. It will have a degenerated yellow to brown appearance. A second piece of dressing is placed over this degenerating first piece without removing it. The outer bandage is replaced with the next dressing change, four to seven days later. After two to three applications of ECM dressing, no new dressings are added. Typically, a granulation tissue bed is present with the presence of a site-specific matrix that will guide the healing of the wound with tissue like that in the surrounding area. Wound management is continued with appropriate bandaging of the granulating wound as healing progresses.

Secondary-intermediate layer

The main function of the secondary bandage layer is absorption. Thus, it should have good capillarity properties to provide for the collection of blood, serum, exudate, debris, bacteria, and enzymes from the wound. Additional functions of the secondary layer are to pad and protect the wound from trauma, prevent movement, and hold the primary layer against the wound.

Materials that can be used for the secondary layer include specific loose-weave absorbent wrap materials, cast padding, and absorbent bulk roll cotton. One author (SFS) prefers to use the first of these as the secondary layer for bandaging wounds. The latter two have the advantage that it is difficult to apply them too tightly because they tear under low levels of extension. However, they have the disadvantage that if they contact a wound surface, they can adhere to it and be left unrecognized as the bandage is removed. This leaves foreign material on the wound surface. Self-adherent gauze roll or tubular gauze can be placed over the secondary wrap as part of the intermediate layer to provide support and rigidity.

This layer should be applied in a wrapping fashion with about 50% overlap of layers. When wrapping a limb, the wrapping should progress from distal to proximal. The secondary layer should be applied with enough pressure to hold the primary layer in contact with the wound and to have good contact between it and the primary layer. However, excessive compression when applying this layer should be avoided since it could impair absorption, blood supply, and wound contraction.

The bandage should be changed frequently (at least daily) on heavily draining wounds to remove exudate that has been absorbed into the secondary layer. Bandage change should be before exudate soaks through to the tertiary layer. This could result in exogenous bacteria wicking inward toward the wound. To help prevent this potential for wound contamination, antimicrobial gauze roll can be used as the secondary layer. When less fluid is absorbed into the secondary layer (e.g., with use of an MRD or as healing progresses), the secondary layer bandage is changed less often.

Tertiary-outer layer

This layer's main function is to hold the other bandage layers in place and protect them from external contamination. Materials that are used for this layer are porous surgical adhesive tape, occlusive waterproof tape (e.g., duct tape), elastic adherent or self-adherent material, and stockinette.

When applying this layer, certain factors should be kept in mind. First, the tertiary layer should be applied under the proper tension. It should hold the primary layer in contact with the wound and the secondary layer in contact with the primary layer.

Second, care should be taken that it is not applied too tightly. This can limit the absorption of the secondary layer. In addition, overtight application on the head and extremities can result in respiratory and circulatory problems, respectively. To help prevent this, one author (SFS) applies porous surgical adhesive tape and occlusive waterproof tape as pretorn strips, rather than rolling the tape directly off of the roll onto the bandage. Each strip is applied with about 1/3 to 1/2 width overlap with the previous strip. For application of the elastic tapes, the tape is applied off of the roll. To reduce the danger of applying it too tightly, the tape is secured near the bandage with one hand while pulling it off of the roll. Another guideline for applying the tape is to apply it so that the textured pattern of the tape is distorted but still visible.

A third factor to keep in mind is the occlusiveness of this layer. Porous tape allows fluid evaporation and promotes dryness, which can impede bacterial growth. However, if this layer gets wet, bacteria can wick inward toward the wound. When an occlusive waterproof tape is used, it protects the underlying bandage from exogenous fluid, but it may also lead to excess moisture retention and the need for more frequent bandage changes. This is particularly true of paw bandages in which sweat from the pads in addition to wound exudate results in considerable moisture. It should also be remembered that any fluid that gets into a bandage covered with waterproof tape remains in the bandage.

Other forms of protection are available to hold bandages in place and protect them. These include premade dressing holders, which are breathable, nonwoven polypropylene fabric with Velcro fasteners. They are washable, reusable, and nonconstrictive. They are available in different sizes for the elbow, hip, shoulder, head, abdomen, thorax, and legs. Lycra body suits provide a breathable bandage cover for bandages on the thorax, abdomen, and limbs.

Special considerations in bandaging, casting, and splinting

Frequency of changes

With bandages, the frequency of bandage changes decreases as wound healing progresses. During the early stages of healing when exudate production is greatest, wound observation is very important, and strike-through prevention is necessary, frequent bandage change may be indicated. However, with MRDs that support autolytic debridement, bandages may be left in place up to three days. Conversely, dressings with high absorptive capacity (e.g., gauze) may need to be changed at least daily and possibly more often, depending on the amount of exudate production.

Once a healthy bed of granulation tissue is present and exudate levels are low, the time between bandage changes is expanded. With nonadherent simiocclusive dressings, the time may be extended to three or four days. With some of the other MRDs, the time may be expanded to five to seven days between bandage changes.

There are times when unscheduled bandage, cast, or splint changes are necessary. These include when there has been slippage, strike-through, wetness, external contamination, and damage to the bandage, cast, or splint. Odor, swelling, or hypothermia of tissues adjacent to the bandage (e.g., digits left exposed from a limb/paw bandage) and constant licking or chewing at a bandage, cast, or splint are also indications for a change.

Security

For a bandage, cast, or splint to be effective, it must be secured in place. Security is a challenge in that animal conformation is quite variable (e.g., a chihuahua vs. a great dane), and tolerance of a bandage, cast, or splint can vary between animals. In the following chapters, application of bandages, casts, and splints will be covered to include techniques to help assure security of these applications. Based on the above-mentioned variables, the veterinarian or veterinary technician may need to occasionally modify a technique and use it in combination with some type of restraint to maintain a secure bandage, cast, or splint. However, if a modification is done, an adage should be remembered: "First, do no harm." Sound clinical judgment is important in applying bandages, casts, and splints.

Pressure relief

Prevention of pressure from bandages, casts, and splints is important from two standpoints. First, there must be prevention of pressure-induced injury from a bandage, cast, or splint being placed too tightly. This is particularly important in placing bandages on extremities and the head, especially when elastic taping material is used. Techniques for helping prevent such pressure are described in sections of this book (see pages 4–9 in chapter 1, Bandaging, Components of a Bandage, and Tertiary-Outer Layer; all of chapter 2; and page 56 in chapter 4, Basic Paw and Distal Limb Bandage).

The second important factor in pressure relief is prevention of localized pressure wounds over prominences caused by a bandage, cast, or splint and prevention of paw pad wound pressure. Techniques for prevention of such wounds are described in sections of this book (see, in chapter 4, Forelimb Bandages, Casts, and Splints; Basic Soft Padded Limb Bandage [pg. 47]; Basic Paw and Distal Limb Bandage [pg. 56]; Paw Pad Pressure Relief [pg. 69]; Carpal Sling [pg. 75]; Spica Bandage and Lateral Splint [pg. 83]; Aluminum Rod Loop Elbow Splint [pg. 88]; and 90/90 Sling [pg. 104]).

Joint immobilization

Wounds over joints can have problems in healing due to joint movement. Thus, joint immobilization is indicated for optimal healing. Such immobilization is attained with a bandage, cast, or splint.

A wound over the extension surface of a joint is subject to separation of the wound edges as the joint is flexed (fig. 1.2). In a sutured wound, the tension of joint flexion could result in sutures pulling out of tissues. Thus, wound immobilization is indicated.

With a large open wound on the flexion surface of a joint, open wound healing could result in wound contraction ending in a wound contracture deformity, whereby the joint is pulled into a flexed position and cannot be extended (fig. 1.3). Immobilizing the joint in extension may help prevent this deformity. The wound may heal mainly by epithelialization and may need a skin graft or flap for a more durable cover, but contracture deformity has been avoided.

Prolonged joint immobilization may lead to disuse atrophy, joint stiffness, pressure wounds, and cartilage degeneration. At bandage changes, the clinician should not only care for the wound but also evaluate joints for problems.

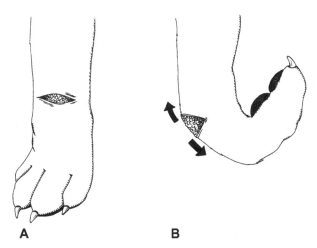

A   **B**

Fig. 1.2.   Wound disruption with flexion. (A) Wound over the extension surface of the carpus. (B) Carpal flexion results in separation of wound edges (arrows).

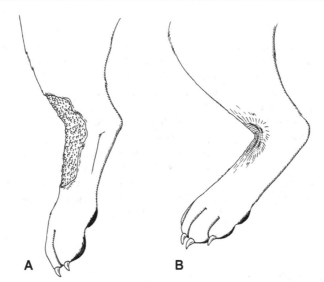

Fig. 1.3.   Wound contracture with open wound healing. (A) Large wound over flexion surface of the hock. (B) Open wound healing with wound contraction, resulting in wound contracture deformity with limited hock extension.

Maceration and excoriation

Maceration is basically overhydration of skin around a wound. It is caused by prolonged contact of the skin with wound exudate. This compromises the skin's barrier function.

Excoriations are skin abrasions caused by high levels of matrix metalloproteinases (enzymes) in exudate of chronic wounds. These also compromise the barrier function of the skin.

A contact bandage layer should be chosen that is appropriate for the amount of exudate being produced by the wound. In this way, a large amount of exudate is not held over the wound to cause maceration and excoriation. To help prevent maceration and excoriation when using MRDs, the dressing can be cut to the size and shape of the wound so that it does not overlap onto healthy surrounding skin.

Need for sedation or anesthesia during bandage change

There are several ways to decrease the pain and discomfort associated with bandage changes. Autolytic debridement with nonadherent MRDs is less painful than the mechanical debridement that occurs with adherent wet-to-dry and dry-to-dry dressings. However, if the latter dressings are used, the last layer of gauze in contact with the wound can be moistened with warm 2% lidocaine for a few minutes before it is removed to provide comfort. In cats, warm physiologic saline is used for this purpose. To remove adhesive tape from the skin, it should be removed in the direction of hair growth, with counter traction provided by a hand on the skin. Ethanol or commercial adhesive remover can also be used to loosen adhesives. To prevent epidermal stripping when tape is removed from the skin, a hexamethyldisiloxane solution can be applied to the skin before applying the tape.

For some animals, sedation may be required for bandage changes, especially during early wound management when staged debridement and lavage are being done. Although there may be additional expense and risk with sedation, the animal is more tractable, wound management is accomplished better, and there is less stress on the animal and personnel. General anesthesia may be needed for aggressive surgical debridement and for bandage changes when a wound is painful or an animal is particularly aggressive.

Casts and splints

General information

Cast and splints rely on many of the same materials and layers used in other types of bandages, with a few exceptions. Generally, cast padding, gauze and various outer layers all provide the same purposes and are used in the manner described for each casting and splinting procedure. Because casts and splints may be in place for a prolonged period, and because they have an inflexible component, the need to prevent pressure wounds is critical. However, paying close attention to avoiding wrinkles, pressure on anatomic prominences, and motion within the cast or splint is also very important.

Purposes and functions of casts and splints

The materials that set a cast or splint aside from other bandages are those that provide a degree of rigidity. The purpose may be to stabilize a fracture in order to allow boney union or merely to allow more comfortable transport of the animal. Splints and casts may protect surgical repairs or support soft tissue injuries. The rigidity of a cast will exceed that of a splint, and an intact cast provides more support than one that has been split ("bivalved") and then reapplied. The rigidity may be achieved through the use of aluminum splint rods, commercial plastic and metal splints, plaster casting tape, fiberglass casting tape, or other materials that are of suitable size and stiffness, such as thermomoldable plastic.

Materials

Splint rods

Splint rods are inexpensive, but they do not conform as well to the limbs as fiberglass tapes. They must be cut and bent to shape. Care should be taken to assure that the cut ends do not injure the animal.

Commercial splints

Commercial plastic and metal splints are available in a variety of sizes and shapes. Some will work better than others depending on the patient, location, and need. Generally, it is best to keep a variety of brands and sizes on hand in order to determine which will work best for a given case. The metal splints (e.g., Mason metasplints) can be cut with metal cutting shears to modify them if needed. Splints should be applied after a basic bandage is applied (i.e., a bandage consisting of a contact layer, cast padding as secondary bandage wrap, and gauze wrap) and then fixed to the limb with a nonelastic material such as porous adhesive tape.

Plastic splinting material

Thermomoldable plastic materials are available for molding splints. These are heated in hot water and are then manually molded to the conformation of the area being splinted. The materials can also be cut with shears when they are in their heated state. When cooled, they return to a rigid state.

Stockinette

Placing stockinette beneath casting material is not absolutely necessary, but it seems to help provide some degree of comfort in the authors' opinion. When stockinette is applied longer than a cast, it can be folded back onto the cast to roll a small amount of cast padding over the edge of the cast to create a soft "bumper" that will protect the tissue from the sharp edge of the cast.

Casting tapes

Casting tapes can be used to make a custom splint or a full cast. Fiberglass tape is preferable to plaster because it is light, durable, and water resistant. However, plaster is inexpensive and sets more slowly and at a lower temperature. When using fiberglass tape, care should be taken to avoid stretching the tape during application because it will slowly return to its original length. In a splint application, this will result in a splint that is too short. In a cast application, it will result in a cast that is too tight.

2 Head and Ear Bandages

Emergency ear bandage

Indications

The most common use of the emergency bandage is in hunting/working dogs that sustain a laceration of the pinna from a thorn or barb on a barbed wire. By instinct, the dogs shake their head to try to rid themselves of the irritation of the ear laceration. The head shaking further irritates and injures the pinna and splatters blood on the dog's surroundings. The emergency ear bandage is indicated to immobilize the injured pinna against the dog's head to prevent further injury to the pinna and to prevent the dog from splattering blood on its surroundings.

Technique

- A section of a leg from a pair of pantyhose is cut such that it is the approximate length of the dog's head. This can be kept in a first aid kit to be taken to the field with the dog. A section of orthopedic stockinette could also be used.
- When it is indicated, the section of the pantyhose leg can be pulled over the dog's head to immobilize the ear against the head (fig. 2.1).

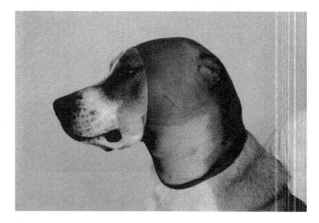

Fig. 2.1.

Samll Animal Bandaging, Casting, and Splinting Techniques   Steven F. Swaim, Walter C. Renberg, and Kathy M. Shike
© Steven F. Swaim, Walter C. Renberg, and Kathy M. Shike

Aftercare

If the dog persists in head shaking and the pantyhose segment tends to slip back, it may be necessary to tape the front edge of the pantyhose segment circumferentially around the dog's head. A piece of 2-inch (5 cm)-wide adhesive tape is used. Half of the width of the tape goes on the hair/skin of the head and the other half is on the front edge of the pantyhose.

Advantages and complications

The emergency ear bandage is small and easily carried in a field first aid kit. It is readily available and quickly applied in the field. It provides protection for the ear until more definitive care can be administered to the ear.

Basic head and ear bandage

Indications

The basic head and ear bandage is indicated for protection of wounds in this area. This includes wounds associated with correction of auricular hematomas, total ear canal ablation, trauma, or tumor removal.

Technique

The following is a description of the technique for placing a head and ear bandage on a dog that has had surgery on the pinna (e.g., auricular hematoma correction) and needs to have medication placed in the ear canal. The same bandage would be used for treatment of other conditions, except that the aperture for applying ear medication would not be cut.

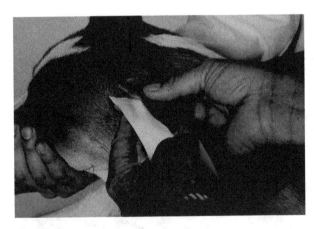

Fig. 2.2.

- To help assure adhesion of tape to the pinna of the ear for applying "stirrups," both the convex and concave sides of the pinna should be shaved, scrubbed, and allowed to dry.
- "Stirrups" are placed on the rostral and caudal edges of the ear. A strip of 2-inch (5.0 cm)-wide adhesive tape that is long enough to wrap around the dog's head is used. The strip is aligned parallel with the long axis of the pinna along the rostral edge of the ear on the concave surface of the ear, with the adhesive surface against the ear. One half of the width of tape is against the ear (fig. 2.2).

- The other half of the tape width is folded over onto the convex surface of the rostral edge of the ear. This sandwiches the rostral edge of the ear between the two layers of tape with the rostral edge of the ear in the fold of the tape (fig. 2.3).
- The length of tape beyond the distal end of the ear is folded over on itself to form a 1-inch (2.5 cm)-wide "stirrup".

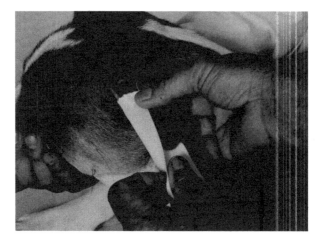

Fig. 2.3.

- This procedure is repeated on the caudal edge of the ear to provide two "stirrups" that will be used to hold the ear over the top of the dog's head (fig. 2.4).

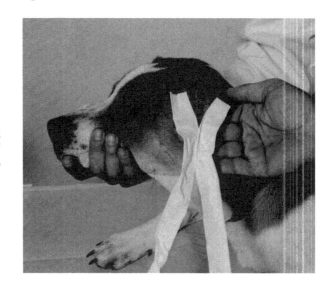

Fig. 2.4.

- A bolus of cotton or a thick pad of cast padding is placed on top of the dog's head at the base of the ear (fig. 2.5).

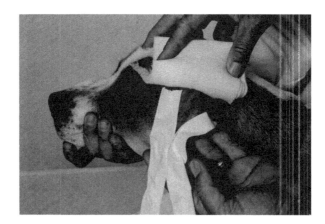

Fig. 2.5.

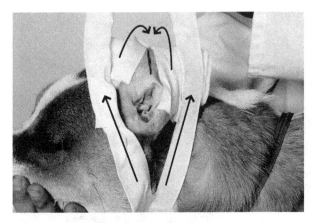

Fig. 2.6.

The two "stirrups" are used to pull the pinna up and fold it over the bolus/pad. The "stirrups" are wrapped around the dog's head (curved arrows) and pulled up in front and in back of the ear that is being bandaged (straight arrows). This leaves the opening of the ear canal open. If auricular hematoma correction surgery has been done, the incision line is between the "stirrup's"attachment on the pinna (dark line; fig. 2.6).

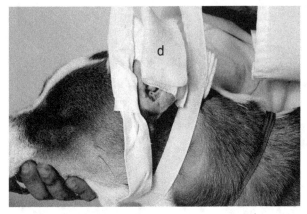

Fig. 2.7.

An appropriate primary dressing is placed over the incision site (d; fig. 2.7).

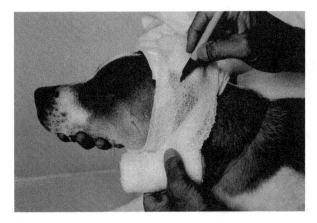

Fig. 2.8.

A roll of secondary bandage wrap is used to wrap the dog's head circumferentially. Each time the wrap goes over the ear canal opening, the location of the opening is marked with a marking pen (fig. 2.8).

Each time a wrap is made with the secondary wrap, it alternately goes in front and in back of the contralateral ear (unoperated ear). When the secondary wrap is completed, the location of the ear canal has been marked (black spot) and the opposite ear is outside of the bandage (being held up; fig. 2.9).

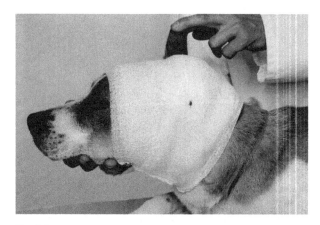

Fig. 2.9.

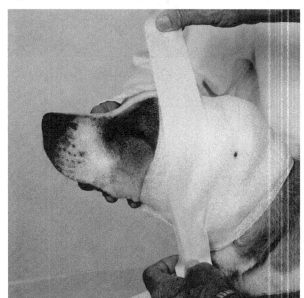

Fig. 2.10.

Pretorn strips of 2-inch (5.0 cm)-wide adhesive tape are placed circumferentially over the secondary wrap (fig. 2.10), and the location of the ear canal opening is marked on the strip that goes over this area (fig. 2.11).

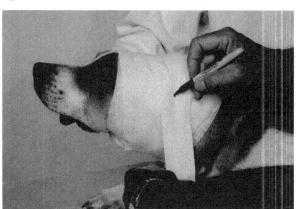

Fig. 2.11.

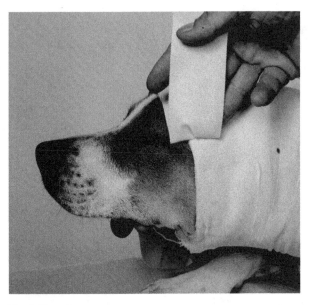

Fig. 2.12.

- A very important strip of tape is placed at the front edge of the bandage. It is placed such that half of the tape's width is on the hair/skin of the head and half is on the bandage (fig. 2.12).
- A similar piece of tape can be placed at the back edge of the bandage to further secure it and keep it from slipping forward, especially on an obese dog with a large neck.

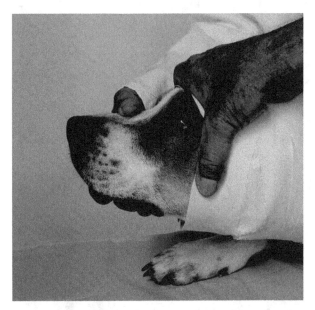

Fig. 2.13.

- After placing this last tape strip, a hand is placed over the strip for approximately one minute. The heat of the dog's body and the heat of the hand help make the tape's adhesive material adhere to the skin/hair for bandage security (fig. 2.13). On small dogs and cats, the distance between the lateral canthus of the eye and base of the ear is short. Thus, use of 1-inch (2.5 cm)-wide tape to fashion the front portion of the bandage may be necessary.

A marker is used to draw a square around the dot marking the location of the ear canal opening. A razor or scalpel blade is used to incise the tape layer of the square while leaving the underlying layers uncut (fig. 2.14).

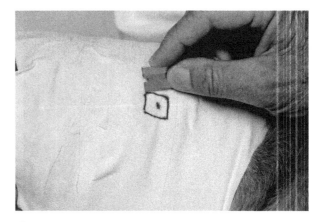

Fig. 2.14.

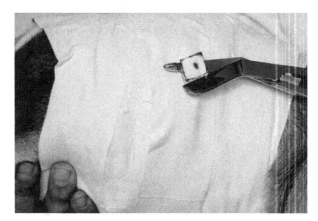

Fig. 2.15.

Bandage scissors are used to remove the square of tape and underlying secondary wrap. (fig. 2.15). This exposes the opening of the ear canal (fig. 2.16).

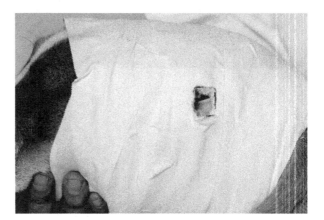

Fig. 2.16.

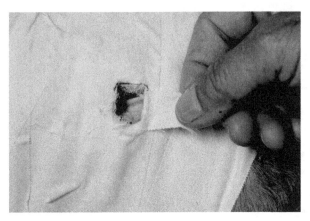

Fig. 2.17.

- Each edge of the square is taped with a strip of 1-inch (2.5 cm)-wide adhesive tape to prevent lint/pieces of secondary wrap from getting into the ear canal (fig. 2.17). It is obvious that the ear is bandaged over the top of the dog's head when an opening has been made over the opening of the ear canal—an important factor during bandage removal.

The following is a description of the technique for placing a head and ear bandage on a dog that will not need to have medication placed in the ear canal. Examples would be bandaging the ear over the top of the head, as would be done for a total ear canal ablation surgery, or bandaging the ear down alongside the dog's head, as with bandaging for a wound on top of the dog's head.

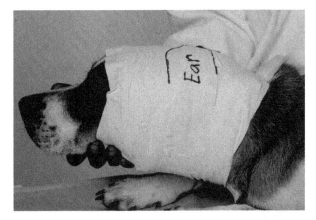

Fig. 2.18.

- When bandaging the ear over the top of the head, the technique for placing the head and ear bandage is as described above, with the exception that marking the location of the ear canal opening on the secondary and tertiary bandage layers and cutting an access hole to this area are not done.
- When bandaging the ear down along the side of the head, no "stirrups" are necessary. A gauze sponge may be placed between the concave ear surface and the side of the head. An appropriate primary dressing is applied to any wound on top of the head. The secondary and tertiary bandage layers are placed as described above. However, the location of the ear canal opening is not marked as these layers are applied.
- After the bandage is in place, a marker is used to draw the location of the ear, either over the top of the head or down along the side of the head. The drawing is labeled "Ear" (fig. 2.18). If a person other than the one who applied the bandage removes the bandage, the labeled ear location helps prevent cutting into the ear at the time of bandage removal.

Aftercare

Protocols for treating auricular hematomas and bandaging the ear and head may vary. The following is that used by the author (SFS). The original bandage is left in place for about seven days. When treatment of otitis externa is associated with the condition, medication can be administered to the ear canal by way of the hole in the bandage over the opening to the ear canal.

At about seven days, the bandage is removed. This is done carefully so as to avoid cutting into the ear that is bandaged over the top of the head. **Thus, cutting the bandage with bandage scissors should be done on the ventral aspect of the bandage** (fig. 2.19), and it should be done carefully so as to leave the "stirrups" intact (fig. 2.20).

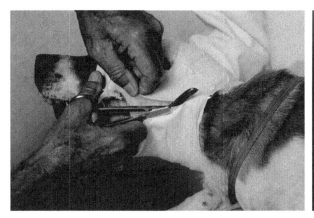 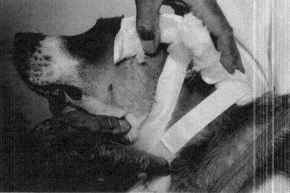

Fig. 2.19.   Removing a head bandage when an ear is bandaged over the top of the dog's head. Cut the bandage on its ventral aspect to avoid cutting the ear.

Fig. 2.20.   The bandage is cut such that the "stirrups" holding the ear over the top of the head are left intact.

The tertiary and secondary layers of the bandage and the primary layer over the surgical site on the pinna are removed. If necessary, the "stirrups" can be unwrapped from around the dog's head. The cotton bolus or cast padding and convex surface of the ear are carefully examined for any moisture. The bolus or pad is replaced and the "stirrups" are rewrapped around the head. The appropriate primary bandage material is placed over the pinna surgical site, and the secondary and tertiary layers are replaced as described for bandage application. This includes making a hole over the ear canal opening for medication application if needed.

Removal and replacement of head and ear bandages is the same for the treatment of conditions other than auricular hematoma. However, appropriate treatment of head and ear wounds is done before bandage replacement.

The author (SFS) uses pretorn strips of white adhesive tape on head and ear bandages. However, elastic bandage material can be used for the tertiary bandage layer. If the bandage is applied while the animal is still anesthetized and intubated, there is danger of getting it on too tight, especially the tertiary layer. When the endotracheal tube is removed, the tight bandage collapses the upper airway, resulting in respiratory embarrassment. Thus, the dog should be observed closely after the endotracheal tube is removed to assure there is no occlusion of the airway, especially if an elastic bandage material was used for the tertiary layer.

Advantages and complications

Head and ear bandages provide good protection for wounds of the head and ears. However, if the front edge of the bandage is not adequately affixed to the hair of the head, the bandage can slip. A dog's first response to the bandage is to try to shake its head and rid itself of the bandage. When this fails, it will try scratching at the bandage with a hind paw. Failure of this leads to the animal's putting its head on the ground/floor and trying to push the bandage back off of its head. If the rostralmost piece of tape on the bandage is not adequately affixed to the hair in this area, the bandage is easily pushed caudally.

3 Thoracic, Abdominal, and Pelvic Bandages

Thoracic, abdominal bandages

Circumferential thoracic, abdominal bandage

Indications

Thoracic and abdominal bandages are indicated to provide covering for wounds on the thoracic and abdominal areas or wounds over the spinal areas of the thorax and abdomen (fig. 3.1). These could be

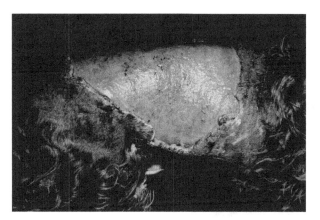

Fig. 3.1. An example of a wound on the thoracic, abdominal, and dorsal spinal areas on which a circumferential thoracic, abdominal bandage would be indicated. Reproduced by permission from Swaim, Steven F., and Henderson, Ralph A., *Small Animal Wound Management*, 2nd ed., p. 155. (Baltimore: Williams and Wilkins, 1997).

Samll Animal Bandaging, Casting, and Splinting Techniques   Steven F. Swaim, Walter C. Renberg, and Kathy M. Shike
© Steven F. Swaim, Walter C. Renberg, and Kathy M. Shike

sutured wounds or open wounds. For sutured wounds, the bandage provides protection of the area from contamination and molestation by the animal. When bandaging an open wound, the bandage not only provides wound protection, but the primary bandage layer can also provide a stimulating effect on the wound healing process. These bandages are especially useful for large wounds over the thoracic and abdominal areas, such as burn wounds.

A basic thoracic and abdominal bandage is also part of using aluminum splint rod side braces (see Side Braces in chapter 5). The bandage is applied prior to placing the side splints. Thus, when the extensions of the side splints are taped in place, they are taped to the bandage and the circumferential body tape wraps are not applied to the hair on the trunk. This makes the presence of the splints more comfortable for the dog.

Technique

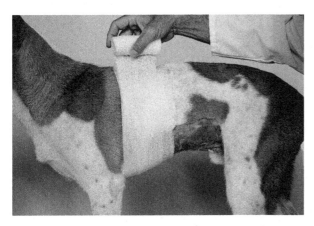

Fig. 3.2.

- When it is indicated (i.e., treating a thoracic or abdominal wound), the appropriate primary bandage layer is placed over the wound.
- Using an absorbent secondary bandage wrap material, the thoracic and abdominal areas are wrapped circumferentially starting on the thorax just behind the forelimbs (fig. 3.2).

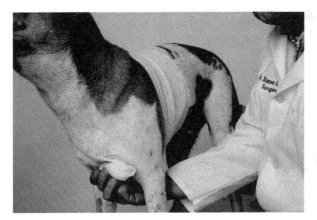

Fig. 3.3.

- After several wraps, the bandage wrapping material is taken up between the forelimbs (fig. 3.3).

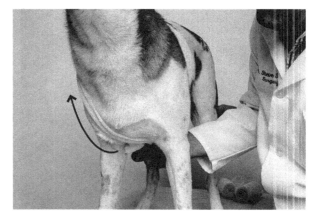

Fig. 3.4.

- The wrap progresses across the pectoral region and up across the opposite shoulder area back onto the front of the body bandage (fig. 3.4 [arrow]). This is done at least two times to give layers of the bandage material across the pectoral area as a strap.

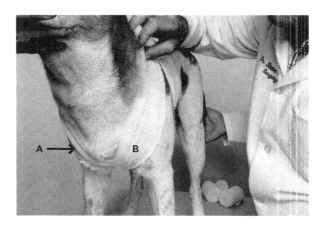

Fig. 3.5.

- This procedure of placing a strap of bandage wrap is repeated on the opposite side. This provides two straps (A and B) of bandage across the pectoral and lower cervical areas that serve as shoulder straps to secure the bandage in place (fig. 3.5).

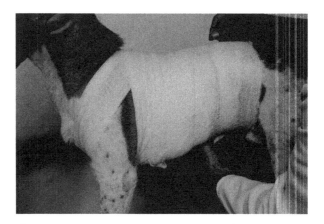

Fig. 3.6.

- After the two straps have been placed, the wrapping of the secondary bandage wrap is continued back onto the abdominal area. Each wrap overlaps the width of the previous wrap by one-half to one-third. Wrapping goes to just in front of the hind limbs. On male dogs, this goes to just in front of the prepuce (fig. 3.6). Two to three layers of wrap are made to cover the thoracic and abdominal areas.

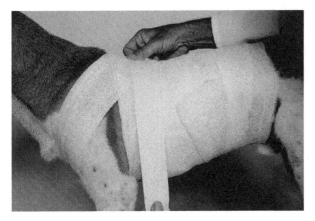

Fig. 3.7.

- Starting just behind the front limbs, pretorn strips of 2-inch (5.0 cm)-wide adhesive tape are placed circumferentially around the trunk to cover the secondary wrap (fig. 3.7). Each strip of tape overlaps the previous strip by one-half to one-third of its width. Alternatively, elastic bandage wrap can be used for this layer.

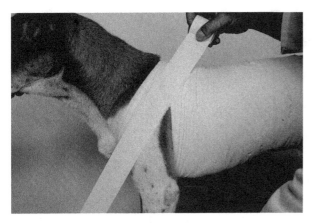

Fig. 3.8.

- Pretorn strips of 2-inch (5.0 cm)-wide adhesive tape are placed over the two straps across the pectoral and lower cervical region. The strips are long enough so that the ends adhere to the body bandage (fig. 3.8). If elastic bandage wrap is used as the tertiary layer, it is used to create the two straps. The completed bandage provides cover for thoracic or abdominal wounds or a bandage surface along which the extensions of side splints can be taped (fig. 3.9).
- To conserve on bandage material, a window can be cut in the bandage over the wound area, and a bandage is placed over this windowed area. This bandage is held in place by tape fixation to the body bandage. Thus, at bandage change, only the bandage covering the wound is changed and the body bandage is left in place unless it has become wet or soiled, in which case it is changed (see page 36 this chapter, Pelvic Bandages, Windowed Pelvic Bandage).

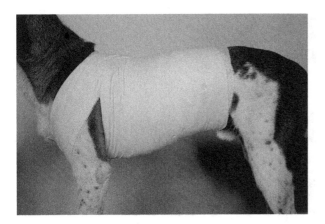

Fig. 3.9.

Aftercare

If daily bandage change is indicated, bandage scissors are used to cut the two shoulder straps and the length of the torso section, and the bandage is removed. The wound is treated and the bandage is replaced. If a windowed bandage is used, the wound is treated through the window and a small bandage is replaced over the window.

The cranial surface of the elbow area should be observed for any irritation that the two shoulder straps might be causing in the area. If this is noticed, a length of gauze can be passed from side to side under the straps and tied. This pulls the straps together and up away from the front of the elbow area.

On male dogs, the preputial area should be observed to check for any skin irritation that the caudal bandage edge may be causing in this area.

Advantages and complications

The bandage provides good coverage for thoracic and abdominal wounds or a good surface on which to fix the extensions of side splints. The shoulder straps provide security and keep the bandage from slipping caudally. If the windowed version of the bandage is used, it conserves on bandage materials since only the portion of the bandage over the wound is changed.

The complication of this bandage is the skin irritation that can be caused by the shoulder straps and the caudal edge of the bandage in the bend of the elbow area and the preputial area on males, respectively.

If a windowed bandage is used, the bandage around the window can become wet and be a source for bacterial growth if wound lavage is used in wound care. Thus, care must be used in cleaning the wound surface.

Windowed thoracic, abdominal bandage

Indications

See page 25 this chapter, Thoracic, Abdominal Bandages; Circumferential Thoracic, Abdominal Bandage. These bandages are indicated for smaller wounds in the thoracic and abdominal areas.

Technique

See page 36 this chapter, Pelvic Bandages, Windowed Pelvic Bandage.

Aftercare

See page 36 this chapter, Pelvic Bandages, Windowed Pelvic Bandage.

Advantages and complications

See page 36 this chapter, Pelvic bandages, Windowed Pelvic Bandage.

Thoracic, abdominal tie-over bandage

Indications

The tie-over bandage can be used to protect open, sutured, or grafted wounds on the thoracic or abdominal areas. The bandage can also be used for the pelvic and proximal limb areas.

Technique

The thoracic or abdominal wound is represented by the fusiform, cross-hatched diagram in figure 3.10.

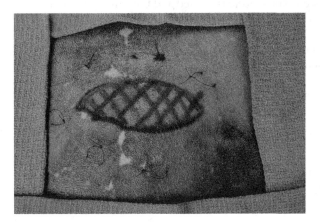

Fig. 3.10.

- Loose loops of 2-0 monofilament suture material (nylon or polypropylene) are placed in the intact skin around the wound (fig. 3.10).

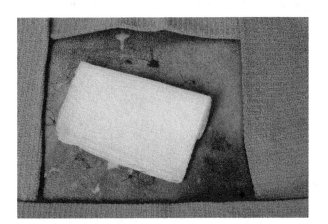

Fig. 3.11.

- The appropriate primary bandage material is placed over the wound (fig. 3.11).

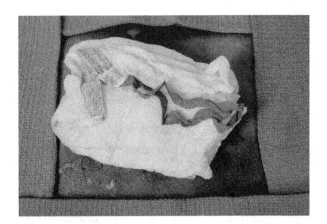

Fig. 3.12.

- A secondary layer of absorbent bandage material (e.g., laporotomy pad) is placed over the primary layer (fig. 3.12).

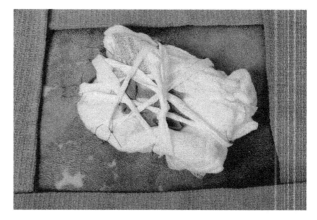

Fig. 3.13.

• A length of umbilical tape or elastic bandage material is laced between the suture loops in whatever pattern holds the bandage layers over the wound best (fig. 3.13).

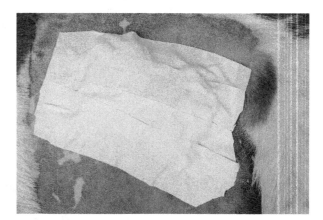

Fig. 3.14.

• Overlapping strips of 2-inch (5.0 cm)-wide adhesive tape are laid over the bandage and adhered to the skin surrounding the wound as the tertiary bandage layer (fig. 3.14). Other impermeable materials could be placed over the bandage.

Aftercare

Frequency of bandage change is governed by the amount and nature of drainage from the wound. At bandage change, the overlying tape strips or impermeable material are removed from the bandage. The umbilical tape or strip of elastic bandage material is cut and removed. The suture loops in the skin are not cut.

• The secondary and primary bandage materials are removed, followed by appropriate wound care.
• Fresh primary and secondary bandage materials are replaced over the wound.
• A length of umbilical tape or a strip of elastic bandage material is threaded through the suture loops around the wound, and tied.
• The tertiary tape strips or impermeable material are placed over the bandage.

Advantages and complications

The main advantage of a tie-over bandage is that it is an economical form of bandage. The large amounts of secondary and tertiary bandage material that are required for a basic thoracic and abdominal bandage are not necessary for a tie-over bandage. The centripetal force from tying the umbilical tape length or elastic strip can be considered as a supplement to wound contraction when treating an open wound.

A potential complication of the tie-over bandage is that the suture loops could cut into the skin if the tie-over strip is tied too tightly. Contamination of the secondary layer of the bandage is possible. However, placing tape or some form of impermeable material over the bandage reduces chances of this complication.

Pelvic bandages

Circumferential pelvic bandage

Indications

The circumferential pelvic bandage is indicated to provide covering for wounds on the pelvic area or wounds over the caudal lumbar and sacral areas (fig. 3.15). These could be sutured wounds or open wounds. The bandage provides protection of the area from contamination and molestation by the animal. When bandaging an open wound, the primary bandage layer can also furnish a stimulating effect on the wound healing process. These bandages are especially useful for large wounds in the pelvic or caudal spinal areas, such as burn wounds.

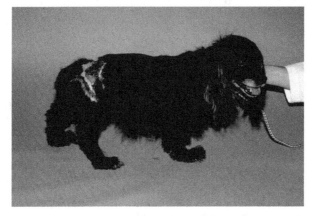

Fig. 3.15.   An example of a wound over the caudal lumbar and sacral area on which a circumferential pelvic bandage would be indicated.

Technique

- The appropriate primary bandage material is placed over the wound.
- Using an absorbent secondary bandage wrap material, the abdominal area is wrapped circumferentially with several layers (fig. 3.16). On male dogs, bandage material is initially wrapped over the prepuce.

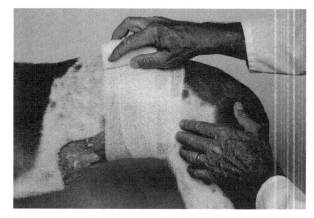

Fig. 3.16.

- Wrapping is continued circumferentially around the proximal aspect of one pelvic limb for two to three wraps (fig. 3.17).

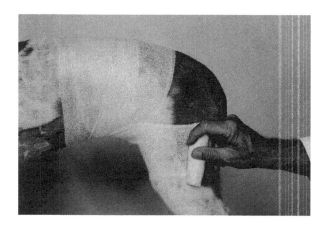

Fig. 3.17.

- The wrapping goes back onto the caudal abdominal portion of the bandage for one to two wraps.
- Wrapping is then taken to the proximal aspect of the opposite pelvic limb where two to three layers of circumferential wrap are made, as with the first limb. On intact male dogs the scrotum should be avoided when wrapping the proximal limbs. The result is a bandage that covers the abdominal, pelvic, and caudal spinal areas, leaving the tail, anus, vulva, or scrotum uncovered (fig. 3.18).

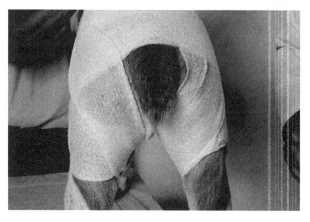

Fig. 3.18.

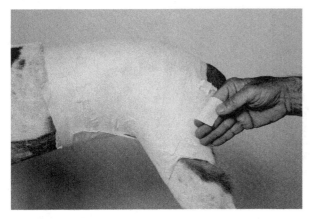

Fig. 3.19.

● Pretorn strips of 2-inch (5.0 cm)-wide adhesive tape are placed over the abdominal and pelvic limb portions of the bandage as the tertiary bandage layer (fig. 3.19). Alternatively, elastic bandage wrap can be used for this layer.

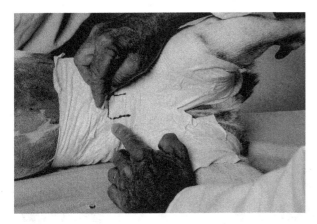

Fig. 3.20.

● On male dogs, the area over the end of the prepuce is marked and a razor blade or scalpel blade is used to cut through the tape layer of the bandage (fig. 3.20).

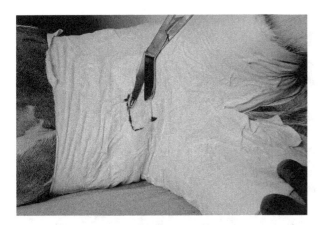

Fig. 3.21.

● Using bandage scissors *carefully*, the secondary bandage material overlying the end of the prepuce is removed (fig. 3.21).

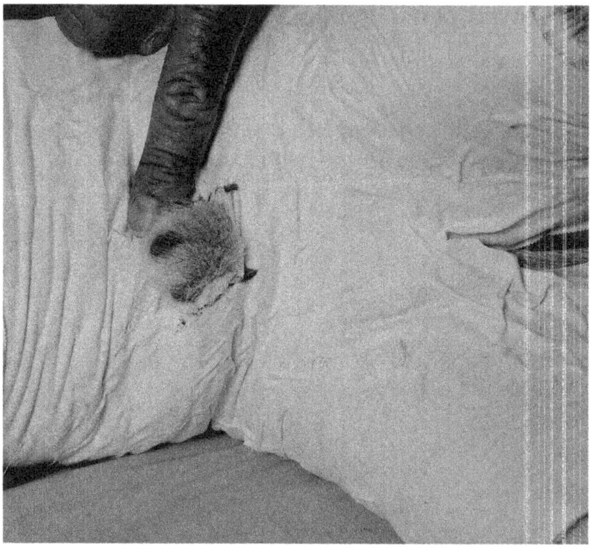

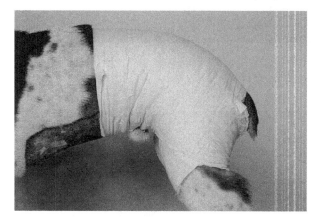

Fig. 3.22.

- The tip of the prepuce is pulled out of the aperture that has been made. If necessary, the scalpel and scissors can be used to extend the opening further cranial to avoid any bandage pressure at the cranial base of the prepuce (the area being pointed out; fig. 3.22). The result is a circumferential pelvic bandage with allowances made for urination and defecation (fig. 3.23).

Fig. 3.23.

Aftercare

If daily bandage change is indicated, bandage scissors are used to cut the bandage along its dorsal surface. The bandage is removed, the wound is treated, and the bandage is replaced.

Advantages and complications

For large wounds, such as burn wounds, in the pelvic and/or caudal spinal areas, these bandages provide an adequate means of keeping medications in contact with the irregular surfaces that are involved. If the preputial opening in the bandage is not large enough, a pressure wound may develop at the cranial base of the prepuce on male dogs.

Windowed pelvic bandage

Indications

See page 32 this chapter, Pelvic Bandages, Circumferential Pelvic Bandage. These bandages are indicated for smaller wounds in the pelvic and caudal spinal areas.

Technique

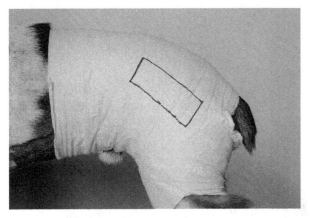

Fig. 3.24.

- A circumferential pelvic bandage is applied (see page 32 this chapter, Pelvic Bandages, Circumferential Pelvic Bandage).
- The area of bandage over the wound is marked (fig. 3.24).

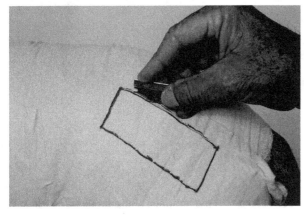

Fig. 3.25.

- A razor blade or scalpel blade is used to incise the tape of the marked area (fig. 3.25).

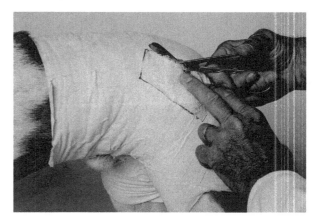

Fig. 3.26.

- Bandage scissors are used to remove the secondary wrap material in the marked area (fig. 3.26). This exposes the wound area (fig. 3.27. No wound is present on this demonstration dog).

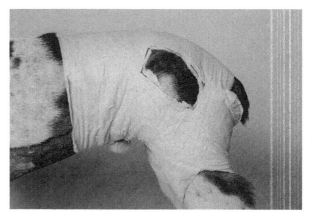

Fig. 3.27.

- Primary and secondary bandage materials are placed over the wound (fig. 3.28).

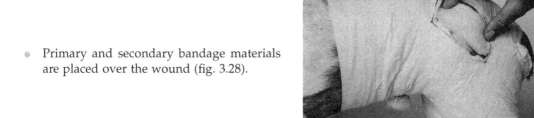

Fig. 3.28.

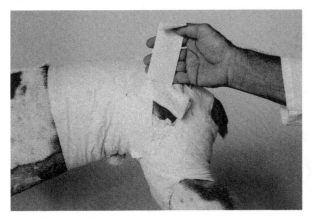

Fig. 3.29.

● Pretorn strips of 2-inch (5.0 cm)-wide adhesive tape are placed over the primary and secondary bandage materials as the tertiary bandage layer to hold them in place (fig. 3.29). These tape strips are adhered to the tape of the circumferential pelvic bandage.

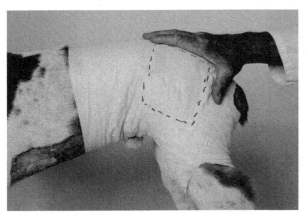

Fig. 3.30.

● A windowed bandage is the result (fig. 3.30. Broken lines indicate tape covering of the windowed bandage).

Aftercare

● At bandage change, the tape of the windowed bandage is removed along with the underlying primary and secondary layers. Appropriate wound treatment is performed.
● Fresh primary and secondary bandage materials are replaced over the wound.
● Pretorn tape strips are placed to hold the underlying bandage materials in place.

Advantages and complications

The main advantage of the windowed bandage is that it is a more economical form of bandage. It is not necessary to replace the entire circumferential pelvic bandage at each bandage change. Only that portion of bandage over the window is changed.

The bandage around the window can become wet and be a source of bacterial growth if wound lavage is used in wound care. Thus, the wound surface must be cleaned carefully to prevent this.

Pelvic tie-over bandage

Indications

See page 29 this chapter, Thoracic, Abdominal Bandages; Thoracic, Abdominal Tie-Over Bandage.

Technique

See page 29 this chapter, Thoracic, Abdominal Bandages; Thoracic, Abdominal Tie-Over Bandage.

Aftercare

See page 29 this chapter, Thoracic, Abdominal Bandages; Thoracic, Abdominal Tie-Over Bandage.

Advantages and complications

See page 29 this chapter, Thoracic, Abdominal Bandages; Thoracic, Abdominal Tie-Over Bandage.

Pelvic extension splints

Indications

Dogs that have had spinal trauma may assume a Schiff-Sherrington posture. They are in a sitting position with the forelimbs extended and supporting the dog's forequarters while the pelvic limbs are extended forward under the dog (fig. 3.31). Thus, the dog's weight is borne on the ischial tuberosities. With side splints that extend beyond the pelvic area, pressure goes on the ends of the splints, keeping it off of the skin over the ischial tuberosities and preventing decubital ulcer formation. The splints are designed for and work best on small dogs (fig. 3.32).

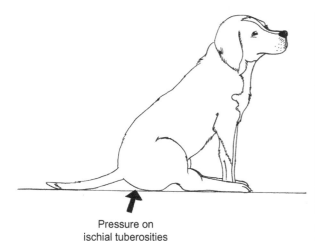

Pressure on
ischial tuberosities

Fig. 3.31.   In the Schiff-Sherrington posture, the dog's weight rests on the ischial tuberosities.

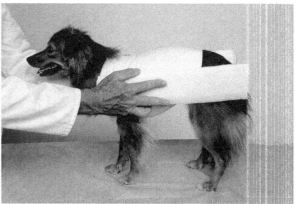

Fig. 3.32.   Pelvic extension splints are designed for and work best on small dogs.

Side splints may also be indicated to protect a tail stump when the tail has been amputated so short that a bandage cannot be applied. They protect the tail stump from pressure as the animal sits.

Technique

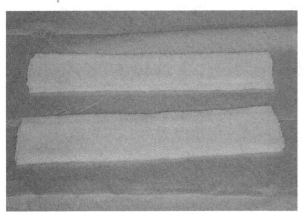

Fig. 3.33.

- A circumferential thoracic, abdominal bandage is placed on the dog (see page 25 this chapter, Thoracic, Abdominal Bandages; Circumferential Thoracic, Abdominal Bandage).
- A rigid splint material that is about 3 inches (7.7 cm) wide is selected for the pelvic extension splints (fig. 3.33).

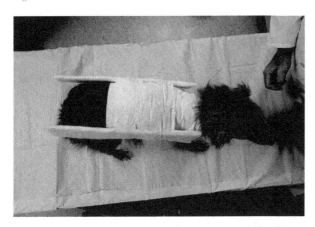

Fig. 3.34.

- The splints are taped on either side of the thoracic, abdominal circumferential bandage with about 2 to 3 inches (7.7 cm) extending beyond the dog's hind quarters (fig. 3.34). When the dog takes the Schiff-Sherrington posture, the caudal ends of the splints take the pressure (closed arrow), not the ischial tuberosities (open arrow, fig. 3.35).

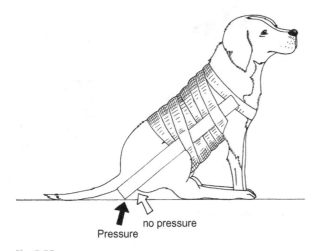

no pressure
Pressure

Fig. 3.35.

Aftercare

The skin over the ischial tuberosities is observed and treated as necessary for the prevention or treatment of pressure wounds. The bandage and splints are adjusted and secured as needed to maintain their function.

Advantages and complications

The splints are an effective method for keeping pressure off of the skin over the ischial tuberosities. This is a major factor in the treatment and prevention of decubital ulcers. They may also be effective in preventing trauma to a short tail stump following tail amputation. The bandage and splints may require adjustment and retaping if they slip. The splints are not as effective on large dogs.

4 Extremity Bandages, Casts, and Splints

Tail bandages

Tail bandages are indicated when there has been an injury to the tail and the wound is being treated as an open wound, a sutured wound, or occasionally as a grafted wound. Bandages provide wound protection and/or protection from pressure on a tail stump.

A common wound of the tail occurs in long-tailed, short-haired dogs that are housed in a kennel environment. When the dog wags its tail, the tip becomes traumatized as it hits against cage or kennel run walls. The result is an open wound on the tip of the tail. A secure bandage is indicated to protect the tail tip while it heals.

When a tail has been amputated at a level such that a bandage can be applied to the remaining stump, a secure bandage is indicated. If the tip of the stump might be traumatized as the animal sits, a splint may be needed to protect the tip of the tail as it heals.

If a tail has been amputated so short that a bandage and/or splint cannot be applied to the stump, side splints may be indicated to protect the stump to prevent molestation and trauma when the animal assumes a sitting posture (see page 39, chapter 3, Pelvic Extension Splints).

Samll Animal Bandaging, Casting, and Splinting Techniques   Steven F. Swaim, Walter C. Renberg, and Kathy M. Shike
© Steven F. Swaim, Walter C. Renberg, and Kathy M. Shike

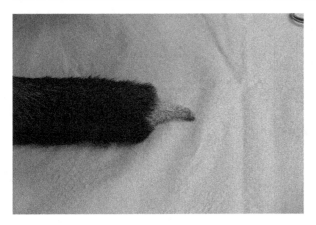

Fig. 4.1.

Technique

- The area proximal to the wound on the tail tip/stump is clipped and prepared for aseptic procedures, especially if any surgical procedure (e.g., suturing) is to be done (fig. 4.1).

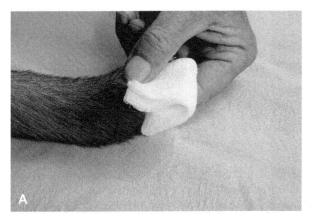

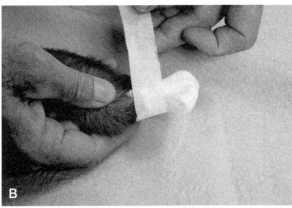

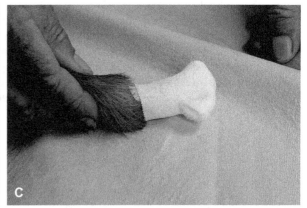

- After applying any necessary medication to the tail stump, a piece of gauze is placed over the stump as the primary dressing and taped in place with a circumferential wrap of 1-inch (2.5 cm)-wide tape (figs. 4.2 A, B, C).

Fig. 4.2.

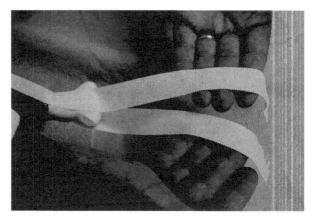

Fig. 4.3.

- Strips of 1-inch (2.5 cm)-wide adhesive tape are placed longitudinally along each side of the tail as "stirrups" (fig. 4.3).

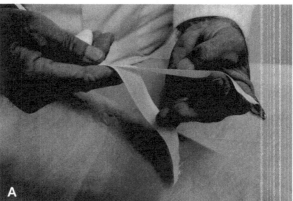

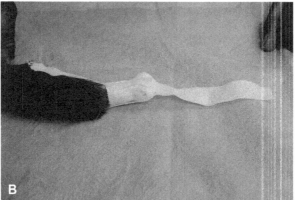

- The tape strips are adhered together beyond the tail tip/stump (figs. 4.4 A, B).

Fig. 4.4.

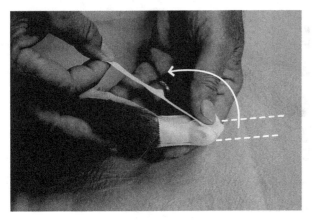

Fig. 4.5.

- The tape strips are folded back onto the tail (fig. 4.5, arrow).

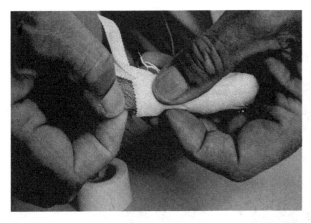

Fig. 4.6.

- Circumferential wraps of pretorn strips of 1-inch (2.5 cm)-wide tape are wrapped around the tail, from distal to proximal. After two or three tape wraps, hair is pulled from beneath the last tape wrap (fig. 4.6).

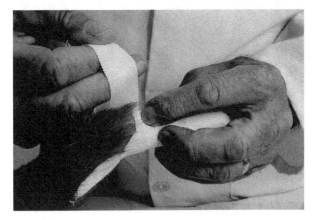

Fig. 4.7.

- The hair thus lies over the last tape wrap and another circumferential segment of the tape is placed to sandwich this hair between its adhesive surface and the nonadhesive surface of the previous tape wrap. This is known as the "shingling" wrap (fig. 4.7).

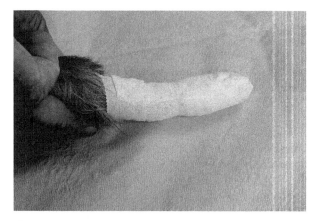

Fig. 4.8.

- The result is a tail bandage secured by tape "stirrups" and "shingling" (fig. 4.8).
- If further protection is needed for a tail stump, an appropriate-sized finger stall–type splint can be taped over the bandage to protect the end of the stump.

Aftercare

The bandage should be kept clean and dry. The frequency of bandage change will depend on the nature of the wound and the clinical judgment of the clinician.

Bandage scissors will be needed to remove the bandage. The "stirrups" and "shingling" technique provides a secure bandage. Thus, removal may require some dilligence.

Because of this, some analgesic/sedation may be needed when manipulating an injured tail to remove the bandage.

Advantages and complications

The primary advantage of the "stirrups" and "shingling" technique is security. The problem with tail bandages is that they can be wagged off, that is, with the centrifugal force of tail wagging, the bandage tends to be thrown off of the tail. "Stirrups" and "shingling" help prevent this.

Because the circulation of the tail becomes more tenuous as the tip of the tail is approached, circulatory compromise could occur if the circumferential tape wraps are placed too tight. To help avoid this, pretorn tape strips are used for these wraps. The danger of getting the wraps too tight is greater if the tape is rolled off of the roll and onto the tail.

Forelimb bandages, casts, and splints

There is some overlap of information about the basic soft padded limb bandage and the basic paw and distal limb bandage. However, some areas require information specific to them. Therefore, to make coverage easier for the reader and thus avoid referring back to areas, a section has been devoted to each topic. Generally, information on the basic soft padded bandage will refer to injuries above the carpus or tarsus, and basic paw and distal limb bandages will refer to injuries from the carpus or tarsus distally. Thus, the reader should refer to both sections if there is concern about what technique to use based on location of an injury.

Basic soft padded limb bandage

This information for the basic soft padded limb bandage on the forelimb also applies to the pelvic limb (see page 92 this chapter, Pelvic Limb Bandages, Casts, and Splints; Basic Soft Padded Limb Bandage).

Indications

The soft padded limb bandage is indicated to provide moderate support, immobilization, and compression to address a variety of needs. It is the fundamental bandage upon which many other techniques are based, such as splints and casts. The bandage is used to protect various soft tissue wounds, such as open wounds, sutured wounds, and grafted wounds.

Technique

Although the pictures shown with this technique are for a forelimb bandage, the principles of the technique are the same for applying the bandage to the pelvic limb.

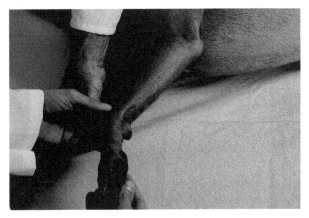

- The animal is generally in lateral recumbency with the affected limb up.
- The limb is placed with neutral angulation of the joints. In most situations, the limb should be maintained in this position while the bandage is applied (fig. 4.9).

Fig. 4.9.

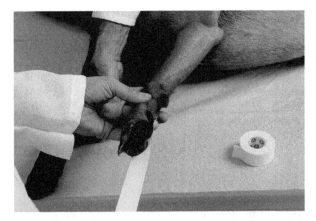

- Tape "stirrups" are applied to the lateral and medial aspects of the paw and metacarpal/metatarsal area using 1-inch (2.5 cm)-wide strips of tape (fig. 4.10).

Fig. 4.10.

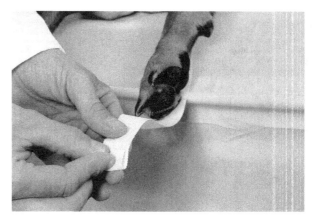

Fig. 4.11.

- The pieces of tape for the "stirrups" should extend beyond the end of the paw 4 to 6 inches (10–15.2 cm). The free end of each piece of tape should be folded over on itself to provide a grip for pulling the strips apart (fig. 4.11). The strips are adhered to each other temporarily (figs. 4.12 and 4.13). Alternatively, a tongue depressor can be placed between the two adhesive surfaces to allow them to be separated. If wounds exist on the lateral or medial aspect of the paw area, the strips can be placed on the dorsal and volar surfaces of the area. There are other techniques for placing "stirrups" for paw wounds (see page 56 this chapter, Basic Paw and Distal Limb Bandage).

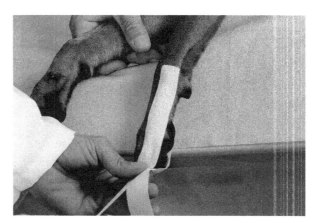

Fig. 4.12.

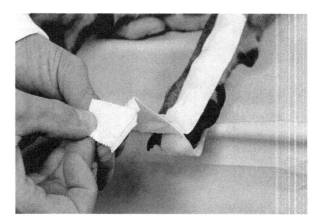

Fig. 4.13.

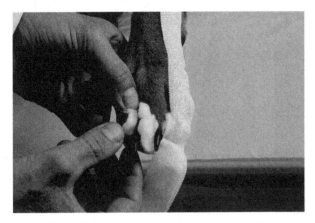

Fig. 4.14.

• Small pieces of cotton or cast padding are placed between the digits and in the interpad area on the palmar/plantar paw surface (fig. 4.14).

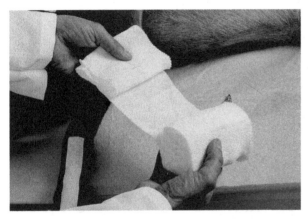

Fig. 4.15.

• The need for protection of the skin over bony prominences or other protrubences (e.g., the carpal foot pad) is assessed so that measures can be taken to prevent pressure wounds. This is especially true if the bandage will be present for a prolonged time, such as under a cast. "Donut" pads can be made by folding several layers of cast padding on each other (fig. 4.15) or by stacking several gauze sponges together to make a pad thick enough to approximate the degree to which the prominence protrudes from the surface of the limb. A hole is cut in the center of the pad to give it the donut effect (figs. 4.16, 4.17, 4.18, 4.19). These pads are placed over the prominences with the hole over the prominence (fig. 4.20). (For an alternative way to make donut pads, see page 56 this chapter, Basic Paw and Distal Limb Bandages).

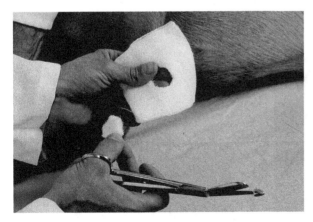

Fig. 4.16.

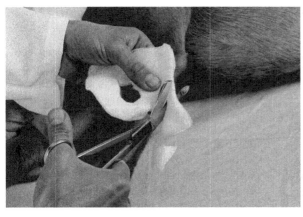

Fig. 4.17.

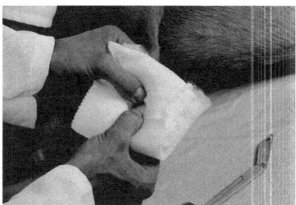

Fig. 4.18.

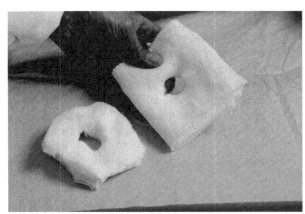

Fig. 4.19.

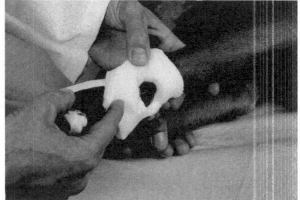

Fig. 4.20.

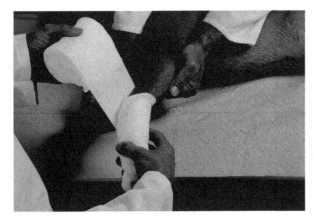

Fig. 4.21.

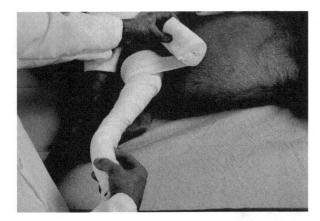

Fig. 4.22.

- If the bandage is to be used for covering a wound or wound repair area, the appropriate medication and primary bandage layer are placed over the wound.
- Cast padding is applied by wrapping the limb from distal to proximal, starting at the digits (figs. 4.21, 4.22). The width of cast padding used is dependent on the size of the animal. Effort should be made to overlap each turn around the limb approximately fifty percent over the preceding turn. Additionally, wrinkles should be avoided, and the material should be stretched to slightly distort the pillow texture if a textured type of cast padding is used. Concern about getting cast padding wrapped too tightly is not a factor since it will tear if too much tension is placed on it.
- If the bandage is being used to cover a draining wound, an absorbent secondary wrap designed to absorb wound fluid is preferred to cast padding. The wrap is applied in the same manner as described for cast padding; however, care must be taken not to wrap it too tightly because it will not tear if excess tension is applied.

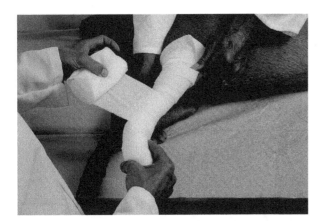

Fig. 4.23.

- At the proximal end of the bandage, tension is evenly applied across the roll of cast padding to tear the roll of padding. Additional layers are commonly applied (figs. 4.23, 4.24).
- When treating a draining wound, several layers of absorbent secondary wrap are applied to absorb wound fluid. The wrap material is cut after sufficient layers have been applied, usually three to four layers.

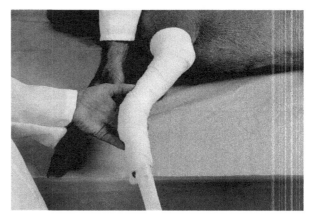

Fig. 4.24.

- The next layer is roll gauze, which is applied from distal to proximal starting at the digits. There should be fifty percent overlap of each wrap with the previous wraps. The gauze should begin and terminate such that a small amount of underlying cast padding protrudes from under it at the top and bottom of the bandage. It is important to apply even tension across the roll during application by keeping fingers on the roll and not on the extended portion of the gauze (fig. 4.25). Tension is applied to supply mild compression of the underlying cast padding. However, excess tension should be avoided because it could inhibit venous and lymphatic return from the limb.
- When the bandage is being used to treat a draining wound, this layer of roll gauze is not used.

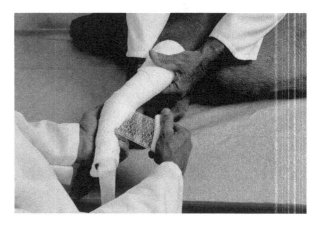

Fig. 4.25.

- The tape strips of the "stirrups" are separated. Each one is twisted so the adhesive side will be against the bandage. They are then folded up onto the bandage. The middle two digits should be visible (fig. 4.26).

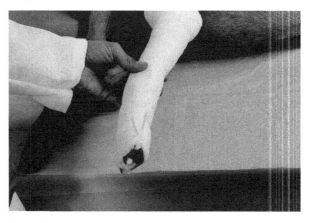

Fig. 4.26.

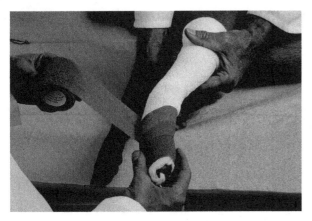

Fig. 4.27.

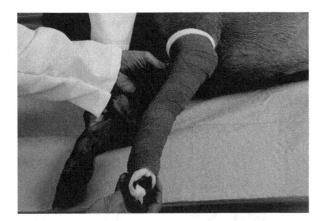

Fig. 4.28.

- The final protective layer can be applied with elastic wrap bandage material. It is applied from distal to proximal with fifty percent overlap of each wrap with the previous wrap and no wrinkles being present (fig. 4.27). It is applied with moderate tension such that the textured pattern of the material is slightly distorted but still visible. There are factors that govern the amount of pressure within an elastic tape outer wrap (see page 56 this chapter, Basic Paw and Distal Limb Bandage). A small amount of the underlying layer should protrude at the top and bottom of the bandage (fig. 4.28).

Alternatively, porous adhesive tape can be used for the outer layer of the bandage. Strips of tape are pretorn before they are applied to the bandage. Each strip is long enough to go once around the bandage circumferentially. The strips are applied from distal to proximal with mild but not constrictive pressure with fifty percent overlap of strips.

Aftercare

The bandage should be carefully monitored. It should be kept clean and dry, and the animal should not be allowed to lick or chew at it. The two exposed digits should be examined for signs of swelling (separation of the digits), which would indicate the bandage is too tight and needs to be changed. A veterinarian should be contacted if the animal's use of the limb decreases or if any of the above signs are noticed.

If the bandage has been used for treating a draining wound, periodic bandage changes will be necessary.

Bandage removal

The bandage should be removed in layers to provide comfort for the animal. The following is the removal technique for a bandage covering a wound. Some of the steps will apply to removing a bandage that underlies a cast or splint being used for orthopedic treatment.

- A razor, scalpel blade, or scissors should be used to carefully cut *only* the tertiary bandage layer for the length of the bandage.
- The tertiary bandage layer is then removed by peeling it away from the underlying layer. If porous adhesive tape was used for the tertiary layer, bandage scissors will be needed to snip the attachment between the two layers.
- An end of the secondary layer is found or created and the secondary layer is unwrapped from the limb. The amount of exudate in the layer should become less with each bandage change as healing progresses. If "stirrups" are present, the position against the skin can be left intact and subsequent "stirrups" applied on top.
- Cotton, cast padding, or primary dressing pieces in the interpad and interdigital areas are removed if they are wet or soiled.
- The primary bandage layer is removed and the wound area is treated appropriately (e.g., debrided, lavaged, medicated). If the primary layer is adhered to the wound surface, it can be soaked with warm physiologic saline or warm 2% lidocaine that does not contain epinephrine. Physiologic saline should be used on cats. This loosens the bandage for removal and provides comfort for the animal.

The layered removal of the bandage is much more comfortable for the animal than trying to manipulate the injured limb and bandage scissors with force to cut through all layers of the bandage at one time.

Bandage replacement

- The pieces of cotton or cast padding are replaced in the interdigital and interpad area if they were removed.
- Depending on the nature of the wound, the appropriate bandage material is replaced over the wound or graft.
- Donut pads can be saved from the previous bandage and be replaced in the new bandage. After two to three uses, these pads become compressed and need to be replaced with new pads.
- If the "stirrups" have become wet with wound drainage, they are replaced.
- The secondary layer is replaced. The amount of exudate being produced will govern the frequency of bandage changes. In the early stages of wound management, when wound fluid production is greatest, bandage changes should be done at least daily. Bandage change should be done before exudate reaches the tertiary layer (strike-through), especially if a porous tertiary layer has been used. If the tertiary layer becomes wet, exogenous bacteria can contaminate the wound. Bandage changes can become less frequent as healing progresses and fluid production decreases.
- The tertiary layer is replaced using either elastic bandage wrap or porous adhesive tape. To help keep the tertiary bandage layers dry and clean, a plastic bag (e.g., bread sack or IV fluid bag) can be placed over the bandage when the animal is in a wet or potentially contaminating environment. Rubber bands should *not* be used to affix the plastic bag on the limb. Tape should be used to secure the bag to the hair above the bandage. Thus, the possibility of the rubber band slipping off of the bag and going unnoticed up under the hair to cause circumferential damage is avoided.

Advantages and complications

The soft padded bandage is easy to apply, and it provides appropriate support and protection for a variety of circumstances. General complications include bandage slippage, pressure wounds, and mutilation of the bandage by the animal. If any of these are suspected, the bandage should be changed. Each area of the bandage has its advantages and complications.

Interdigital and interpad areas
The pieces of cotton or cast padding placed between the digits and interpad area help absorb the normal moisture in the area and help prevent bacterial growth. However, if they get wet they promote bacterial growth.

Primary bandage layer
The advantages and complications associated with the various primary bandage materials are covered in chapter I, Basics of Bandaging, Casting, and Splinting. In general, the newer primary dressing materials enhance the healing process by creating an environment that supports wound healing or by interacting with tissues to enhance healing. The donut pads provide an inexpensive way to protect the skin over convex prominences from pressure injury. The "stirrups" help assure security of the bandage on the limb. However, if they become wet, they may become a source of bacterial growth and wound contamination.

Secondary bandage layer
The absorption of exudate and its associated bacteria away from the wound is the main advantage of the secondary bandage layer. The secondary layer also provides padding and some immobilization of injuries.

When a porous tertiary layer has been used, fluid can evaporate from the exudate, and this helps inhibit bacterial growth. The 0.2% polyhexamethylene biguanide–impregnated secondary dressing has the added advantage of inhibiting wound bacteria and exogenous bacteria that may enter the secondary layer.

With highly productive wounds, evaporation of fluid from the secondary layer may not be as fast as absorption. Thus, wound bacteria and exogenous bacteria may proliferate in the bandage. In such wounds, frequent bandage changes are indicated.

If cotton or cast padding is used in the secondary layer, and if they come in contact with the wounds and become wet, they may stick to the wound. They are difficult to see and thus small amounts are left on the wound and can act as foreign bodies. However, cast padding has an advantage as a secondary layer in that it is difficult to wrap it too tightly. It will tear if too much tension is placed on it while wrapping it.

Tertiary bandage layer
This layer holds the other layers in place. If a porous material is used, it allows evaporation of fluid from the secondary layer, which is beneficial in keeping a bandage dry. However, the porosity also can allow exogenous fluid and bacteria to enter the bandage. Elastic bandage materials provide good conformation of the bandage to the limb, but they have the potential complication that they can cause circulatory problems and tissue necrosis if they are applied too tightly.

Basic paw and distal limb bandage

See page 47 this chapter, Forelimb Bandages, Casts, and Splints.

Indications

Bandages on the distal limb and paw are generally indicated for treating open, sutured, or grafted wounds. For some soft tissue wounds, some form of splint is necessary to prevent tissue movement and/or pressure. Some specific indications will also be stated with portions of the technique.

Technique

Interdigital/interpad areas
These areas must be kept dry, and in the presence of wounds they require a primary bandage dressing.

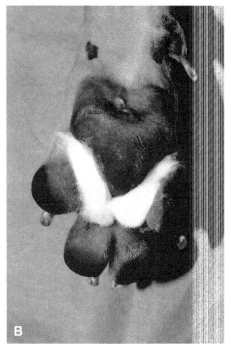

● Small pieces of cotton or cast padding are placed between the digits and in the interpad area on the palmar/plantar paw surface (figs. 4.29 A and B).

Fig. 4.29. From *Small Animal Distal Limb Injuries*, published by Teton New Media (in press).

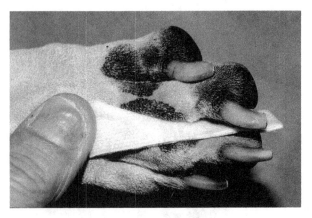

Fig. 4.30. From *Small Animal Distal Limb Injuries*, published by Teton New Media (in press).

●   Alternatively, if there are wounds between the digits, strips of some form of primary dressing should be placed between the digits (fig. 4.30).

Primary bandage layer, "donut" pads, and "stirrups"

The primary bandage layer plays an important role in providing a supportive environment for healing and/or interacting with the wound tissues to enhance healing. Depending on the nature of the wound, the appropriate primary bandage material is placed over the wound or graft (see chapter 1).

"Diapering a paw" is a technique that can be used to apply the primary bandage layer on wounds on the dorsum of the digits or on the pads of medium-sized dogs. It is similar to placing a disposable diaper on a child.

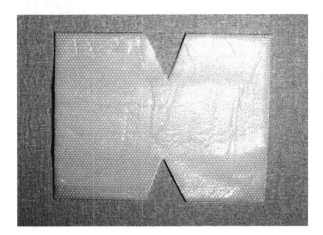

●   Triangular notches are cut from the midpoint along the adhesive edges on either side of a nonadherent semiocclusive pad (fig. 4.31).

Fig. 4.31. From *Small Animal Distal Limb Injuries*, published by Teton New Media (in press).

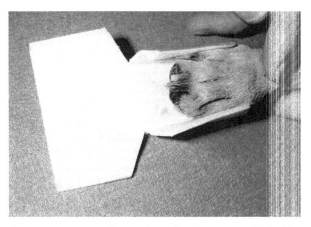

The pad is placed on the palmar/plantar surface of the paw and adhered to the lateral and medial sides of the area (fig. 4.32).

Fig. 4.32. From *Small Animal Distal Limb Injuries*, published by Teton New Media (in press).

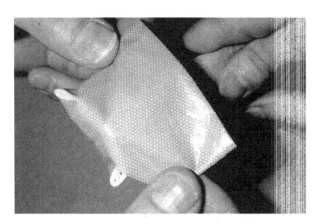

The pad is folded so the remaining portion covers the dorsum of the paw (fig. 4.33).

Fig. 4.33. From *Small Animal Distal Limb Injuries*, published by Teton New Media (in press).

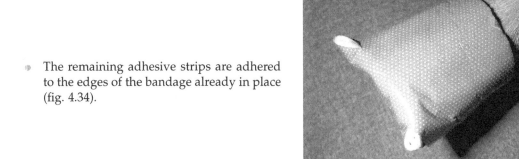

The remaining adhesive strips are adhered to the edges of the bandage already in place (fig. 4.34).

Fig. 4.34. From *Small Animal Distal Limb Injuries*, published by Teton New Media (in press).

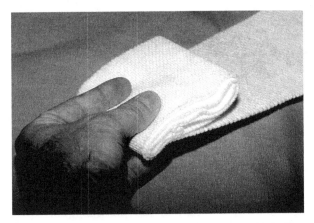

- "Donut" pads are used over prominences such as the carpal pad or the point of the hock that could be injured by bandage, cast, or splint pressure.
- Several layers of cast padding are folded on each other to make a pad approximately 3 inches x 3 inches (7.6 cm × 7.6 cm; fig. 4.35).

Fig. 4.35. From *Small Animal Distal Limb Injuries*, published by Teton New Media (in press).

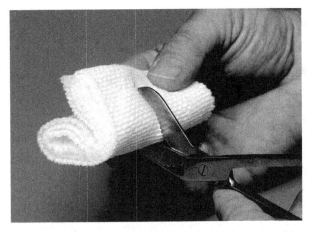

- The pad is folded over on itself, and bandage scissors are used to cut a slit in the center of the pad (fig. 4.36).

Fig. 4.36. From *Small Animal Distal Limb Injuries*, published by Teton New Media (in press).

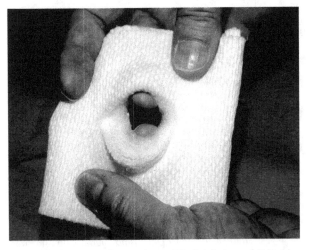

- The pad is unfolded and the slit is enlarged to a nearly round opening using digital tension on its edges (fig. 4.37).

Fig. 4.37. From *Small Animal Distal Limb Injuries*, published by Teton New Media (in press).

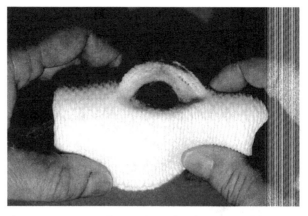

Fig. 4.38. From *Small Animal Distal Limb Injuries*, published by Teton New Media (in press).

🔸 The pad is placed over the prominence with the opening over the prominence (fig. 4.38).

🔸 "Stirrups" can be placed on the limb to help secure a bandage in place.

🔸 Two strips of 1-inch (2.5 cm)-wide adhesive tape are adhered to the skin of the limb parallel to the limb's long axis. Placement of these can be on the dorsal or volar surface (fig. 4.39) or on the medial and lateral surfaces (fig. 4.40). The strips should extend several inches beyond the end of the paw. The placement is dependent on the location of any lesion on the paw or distal limb. "Stirrups" should not be placed over any wound, suture line, or graft. If there is a large wound or graft in the area that would interfere with "stirrup" placement, "stirrups" should not be used.

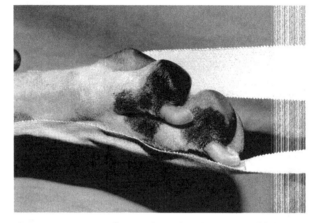

Fig. 4.39. From *Small Animal Distal Limb Injuries*, published by Teton New Media (in press).

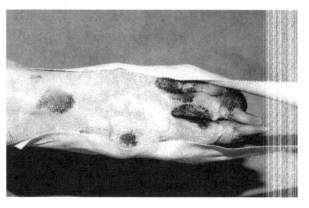

Fig. 4.40. From *Small Animal Distal Limb Injuries*, published by Teton New Media (in press).

Secondary bandage layer

The function of the secondary bandage layer is to provide absorption of wound drainage, padding, and some immobilization. Specific secondary wraps or cast padding can be used (see chapter 1).

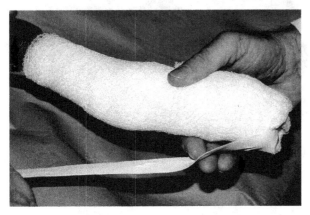

Fig. 4.41. From *Small Animal Distal Limb Injuries*, published by Teton New Media (in press).

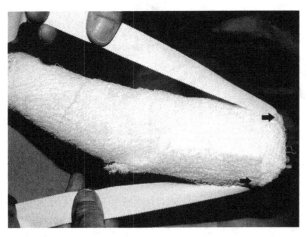

Fig. 4.42. From *Small Animal Distal Limb Injuries*, published by Teton New Media (in press).

- The secondary bandage layer is wrapped onto the limb from distal to proximal. It should be wrapped such that there is good contact between this layer and the underlying primary bandage. However, excess pressure should be avoided. This layer is placed evenly along the limb. The practice of twisting the bandage material 180 degrees to get a narrow portion to pull underlying bandage into an uneven area (e.g., around a carpal paw pad) should not be done. There is increased pressure under such twists.
- Distal end of bandage with "stirrups":

    Option 1—The adhesive surfaces of the "stirrup" strips can be adhered together beyond the end of the paw for 3 to 8 inches (7.6 to 20.4 cm), depending on the length of the bandage/leg. The resulting single strip is folded back onto the secondary bandage surface (fig. 4.41).

    Option 2—Each strip of the stirrup is twisted 180 degrees (arrows) and folded back onto the secondary bandage layer (fig. 4.42). There are other techniques for placing "stirrups"(see page 47, this chapter, Basic soft padded limb bandage).

- Distal end of the bandage without "stirrups": This form of bandaging is especially effective when there are wounds on the digits. It can also be used where the wounds or grafts preclude the use of "stirrups".

  Option 1—At the end of the paw, the secondary bandage roll is turned at a right angle in preparation for placing layers over the end of the paw (fig. 4.43). The bandage material is folded back and forth over the end of the paw several times (fig. 4.44). The bandage roll is then turned at a right angle again and wrapped circumferentially around the paw area to pull in the protruding edges of the folds (fig. 4.45). The result is a smooth bandage enclosing the paw (fig. 4.46).

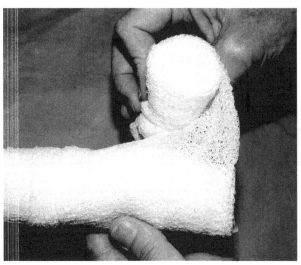

Fig. 4.43.   From *Small Animal Distal Limb Injuries*, published by Teton New Media (in press).

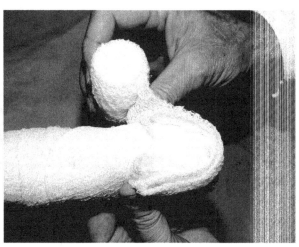

Fig. 4.44.   From *Small Animal Distal Limb Injuries*, published by Teton New Media (in press).

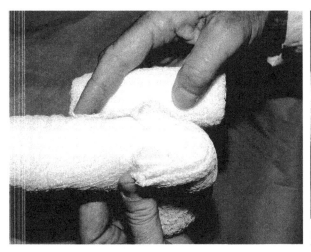

Fig. 4.45.   From *Small Animal Distal Limb Injuries*, published by Teton New Media (in press).

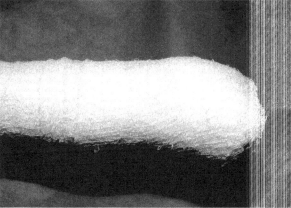

Fig. 4.46.   From *Small Animal Distal Limb Injuries*, published by Teton New Media (in press).

Option 2—Wrapping the secondary roll begins at the level of the second and fifth digits, wrapping obliquely so the third and fourth digits are not covered by the bandage but remain exposed (fig. 4.47). This allows the evaluation of bandage tightness. If the digits appear swollen or feel hypothermic, it is an indication the bandage may be too tight. This option for the distal end of the bandage could be used when the wounds or grafts preclude the use of "stirrups". It can also be used when medial and lateral stirrups are employed, since the digits could remain exposed.

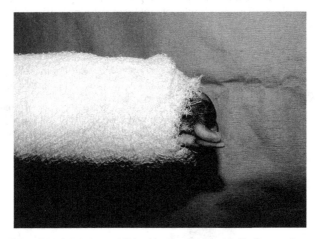

Fig. 4.47.   From *Small Animal Distal Limb Injuries*, published by Teton New Media (in press).

Tertiary bandage layer

This layer secures the other bandage components in place, keeps them clean, and helps immobilize the bandaged distal limb, especially when the layer holds a splint in place. Several materials are available for this layer (see chapter 1).

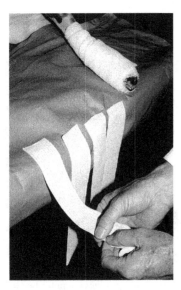

Fig. 4.48.   From *Small Animal Distal Limb Injuries*, published by Teton New Media (in press).

- Tertiary bandage material is placed over the secondary layer.

  Option 1—If porous adhesive tape is used, strips of tape are pretorn before applying them to the bandage (fig. 4.48). Each strip is long enough to go around the bandage circumferentially. Strips of tape are applied from distal to proximal on the bandage, with mild but not constrictive pressure in an overlapping fashion.

- Alternatively, the tape can be rolled off of the roll as it is applied to the bandage. However in doing this, it is necessary to secure the tape near the bandage with one hand while pulling more tape off of the roll. Thus, the danger of applying tape too tightly is reduced (fig. 4.49).

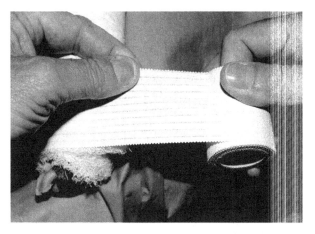

Fig. 4.49. From *Small Animal Distal Limb Injuries*, published by Teton New Media (in press).

- At the proximal end of the bandage, the last piece of tape is placed such that half of its width is on the next-to-last piece of tape and the other half of its width is on the skin at the proximal end of the bandage (fig. 4.50).

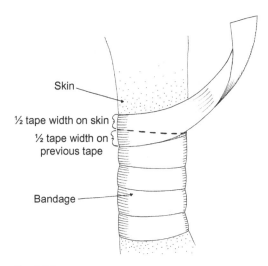

Skin

½ tape width on skin

½ tape width on previous tape

Bandage

Fig. 4.50.

- Additional pieces of tape can be placed to incorporate more skin/hair on the limb at the proximal end of the bandage and thus prevent bandage slippage. A hand can be pressed on the tape over the skin/hair for approximately one minute. The heat of the hand and the animal's body help make the tape's adhesive material adhere to the skin/hair for bandage security.
- Another means to help ensure tape adhesion to the skin is to spray polymeric solution of hexamethyldisiloxane acrylate (Cavilon No Sting Barrier Film, 3M Health Care, St. Paul, MN) on the skin adjacent to the top of the bandage. After drying, it leaves a clear film to which the tape sticks better than only the skin. This film also helps prevent epidermal stripping when the tape is removed.

  Option 2—When waterproof tape is used to protect the bandage from exogenous fluid (e.g., water or urine), it is applied as pretorn strips as described for porous adhesive tape (fig. 4.48). However, it is applied over the porous adhesive tape. Contact of this bandage material with skin and hair on the limb is avoided. Bandage security to the skin and hair is assured by the medical-grade porous adhesive tape.

Option 3—When elastic adhesive tape is applied, it should be done *carefully* over adequate secondary bandage wrap to provide even but *not excessive pressure*. Use of cast padding as the secondary layer can provide relatively more pressure protection when using elastic adhesive tape. As the tape is applied off of the roll, it is secured near the bandage with one hand while pulling more tape off of the roll. Thus, the danger of applying tape too tightly is reduced (fig. 4.49). The wraps should overlap one-third to one-half of the tape width. Another guideline for applying this tape is to apply it such that the textured pattern of the material is slightly distorted but still visible.

When using elastic adhesive tape, it should be remembered that pressure created by this tape is governed by five factors:

1. The material's elasticity. Higher elasticity creates more pressure.
2. The amount of tension placed on the tape during application.
3. The width of the tape. The narrower the tape, the greater the local pressure (tourniquet effect).
4. The number and amount of overlap of layers applied. Pressure is additive with these, that is, each layer may feel as if it is being applied under the correct tension. However, the pressure increases with each layer.
5. The circumference of the bandaged limb. The smaller the circumference, the greater will be the possible pressure (fig. 4.51).

Care should be used when progressing from an area of smaller circumference to one of larger circumference, that is, distal to proximal. The distal portion of the bandage should be applied with less tension to prevent excessive constriction in this smaller circumference area. It should be remembered that there may be some areas that are narrower than more distal areas on some dogs, for example, immediately proximal to the carpus and tarsus and proximal to the digits. A tourniquet effect could result from tight application in these areas. *Adequate padding is important in helping prevent such pressure problems.*

If very convex areas (e.g., point of the hock or point of the elbow) are bandaged with elastic adhesive tape, care needs to be taken to avoid too much pressure. Bandages over these areas normally produce pressure; therefore, elastic adhesive tape has a greater potential for causing excess pressure over the areas. With placement of additional padding over these areas, pressure increases rather than decreases. Thus, it is best to pad around these points with a "donut" pad (see page 58, this chapter, Primary Bandage Layer, "Donut" Pads, and "Stirrups").

To help assess the pressure of a distal limb bandage applied with elastic adhesive tape, the bandage could be applied leaving the middle two digits exposed to be monitored for sensation and circulation

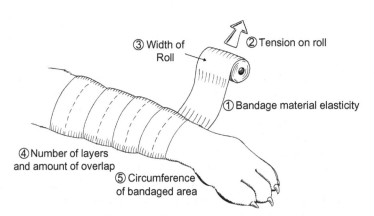

Five Things Governing Banadage Pressure

Fig. 4.51.

several times a day (see page 64, this chapter, Secondary Bandage Layer, Distal End of the Bandage without "Stirrups"—Option 2).

Aftercare

Bandage removal

A distal limb and paw bandage should be removed in layers to provide comfort for the animal. The following is the removal technique for a bandage covering a wound. Some of the steps will apply to removing a bandage that underlies a cast or splint being used for orthopedic treatment.

- Using a razor blade or a scalpel blade, *only* the tertiary layer of the bandage is carefully incised along the length of the bandage.
- At the proximal end of the bandage, where tape of the tertiary layer may be adhered to the skin and hair for security, digital manipulation and bandage scissors are used to release tape attachment.
- The tertiary bandage layer is then removed by peeling it away from the underlying secondary bandage layer. Bandage scissors are used to snip the attachment between the two layers as it is needed.
- An end of the secondary layer is found or created and the secondary layer is unwrapped from the limb. The amount of exudate being produced by the wound can be assessed as this layer is removed. The amount of exudate in this layer should become less with each bandage change as healing progresses. If "stirrups" are present, they are left intact.
- Cotton, cast padding, or primary dressing pieces in the interpad and interdigital areas are removed if they are wet or soiled.
- The primary bandage layer is removed and the wound area is treated appropriately (e.g., debrided, lavaged, medicated). If the primary layer is adhered to the wound surface, it can be soaked with warm physiologic saline or warm 2% lidocaine that does not contain epinephrine. For cats, warm physiologic saline should be used. This loosens the bandage for removal and provides comfort for the animal at removal.

The layered removal of the bandage is much more comfortable for the animal than trying to manipulate the injured limb and bandage scissors with force to cut through all the layers of the bandage at once.

Bandage replacement

- At the time of bandage change, the pieces of cotton or cast padding that have been placed in the interdigital and interpad areas are replaced. If wounds are present in these areas, then pieces of the appropriate primary bandage material are replaced in these areas.
- Depending on the nature of the wound, the appropriate bandage material is replaced over the wound or graft. Diapering the paw may be done if it is indicated, that is, for a wound on the dorsum or palmar/plantar paw surface of the medium-sized dog.
- Donut pads made from cast padding can be saved from the previous bandage and be replaced in the bandage. After two to three uses, these pads become compressed and need to be replaced with new pads.
- If "stirrups" have been used, these are left in place and used in the new bandage. If the "stirrups" have become wet with wound drainage fluid, they should be removed since this would be an area of bacterial growth. The "stirrups" can be replaced or the bandage can be applied without "stirrups". In the latter case, bandage security is dependent on tape fixation to the skin and hair at the proximal end of the bandage.
- The secondary bandage layer is replaced. The amount of exudate being produced will govern the frequency of bandage changes. In the early stages of wound management, when wound fluid production is greatest, bandage changes should be done at least daily. Bandage change should be done before exudate reaches the tertiary layer (strike-through), especially if a porous tertiary layer has been used.

If the tertiary layer becomes wet, exogenous bacteria can contaminate the wound. Bandage changes can become less frequent as healing progresses and fluid production decreases.

- The secondary bandage layer is replaced with appropriate arrangement at the distal end of the bandage, depending on whether "stirrups" have or have not been used.
- The tertiary bandage layer is replaced using either elastic bandage wrap or porous adhesive tape. The tertiary bandage layer should be kept dry and clean. When a porous tertiary layer has been used, a plastic bag (e.g., bread sack, IV fluid bag) can be placed over the bandage when the animal is in a wet or potentially contaminating environment, such as being outdoors for bowel and urinary functions in wet grass. Rubber bands should *not* be used to affix the plastic bag on the limb. Tape should be used to secure the bag to the hair above the bandage. Thus, the possibility of the rubber band slipping off of the bag and going unnoticed up under the hair to cause circumferential damage is avoided.

Advantages and complications

The basic paw and distal limb bandage is easy to apply, and it provides appropriate support and protection for wounds in this area. General complications include slipping, pressure wounds, and mutilation of the bandage. If any of these are suspected, the bandage should be changed. Each area of the bandage has its advantages and complications.

Interdigital/interpad area
The pieces of cotton or cast padding placed in these areas help absorb normal as well as exudative moisture to help prevent tissue maceration and bacterial growth in these areas. With wounds in these areas, the strips of primary bandage material can enhance the healing process.

Primary bandage layer
The advantages and complications associated with the various primary bandage materials are covered in chapter I. In general, the newer dressing materials enhance the healing process by creating an environment that supports wound healing or by interacting with tissues to enhance healing.

Diapering a paw provides a smooth application of a nonadherent semiocclusive pad to the paw of a medium-sized dog if this is the type of dressing that is indicated for the wound.

Donut pads made from cast padding provide an inexpensive way to provide protection for the skin over convex prominences from pressure.

"Stirrups" help assure security of a bandage on the limb. However, if they become wet, they are a source of bacterial growth and wound contamination.

Secondary bandage layer
The absorption of exudate and its associated bacteria away from the wound is the main advantage of the secondary bandage layer. The secondary layer also provides padding and some immobilization of injuries.

When a porous tertiary layer has been used, fluid can evaporate from the exudate, and this helps inhibit bacterial growth. The 0.2% polyhexamethylene biguanide–impregnated secondary dressing has the added advantage of inhibiting wound bacteria and exogenous bacteria that may enter the secondary layer.

With highly productive wounds, evaporation of fluid from the secondary layer may not be as fast as absorption. Thus, wound bacteria and exogenous bacteria may proliferate in the bandage. In such wounds, frequent bandage changes are indicated.

If cotton or cast padding is used in the secondary layer, and if they come in contact with the wound and become wet, they may stick to the wound. They are difficult to see and thus small amounts are left on the wound and can act as foreign bodies. However, cast padding has an advantage as a secondary layer in that it is difficult to wrap it too tightly. It will tear if too much tension is placed on it while wrapping it.

Tertiary bandage layer
This layer holds the other layers in place. If a porous material is used, it allows evaporation of fluid from the secondary layer, which is beneficial in keeping a bandage dry. However, the porosity also can allow exogenous fluid and bacteria to enter the bandage. Elastic bandage materials provide good conformation of the bandage to the limb, but they have the potential complication that they can cause circulatory problems and tissue necrosis if they are applied too tightly.

Paw pad pressure relief

Indications

Wounds of the digital and metacarpal/metatarsal pads can be lacerations, abrasions, punctures, burns (thermal or chemical), or result from tumor removal. Such wounds have special requirements for adequate healing. Pressure and movement of pad tissues must be minimized or prevented. Since pads act as shock absorbers, weight bearing on the pads results in tissues of a wound moving apart as pressure is applied or in sutures tearing through tissue if the wound has been sutured. This impedes healing. Thus, techniques are necessary to relieve pressure in bandaging whether the wound is a simple laceration or a more complicated pad graft. Some specific indications will be stated with portions of the Technique sections.

Technique—moderate wounds on small to medium-sized dogs

Metacarpal/metatarsal pad
A foam sponge "donut" pad can be used for paw pad pressure relief on small to medium-sized dogs that have moderate pad wounds, such as sutured wounds or small open wounds.

- A piece of medium compressibility (blue color) foam sponge padding (Confor™foam, HiTech Foam, Lincoln, NE) is cut to the size and basic shape of the palmar/plantar surface of the paw. The foam pad thickness is split in half using a razor blade or number 10 scalpel blade. Thus, the pad is approximately 0.5 inch (1.25 cm) thick. Using the blade, a hole is cut in the area of the pad that will be over the metacarpal/metatarsal pad wound. Thus, a donut pad is created.
- The primary and all but the last two or three wraps of the secondary layer of a basic paw and distal limb bandage are applied (see page 56 this chapter, Basic Paw and Distal Limb Bandage).
- The donut foam sponge pad is placed on the palmar/plantar surface of the bandage with the hole over the metacarpal/metatarsal pad (fig. 4.52).

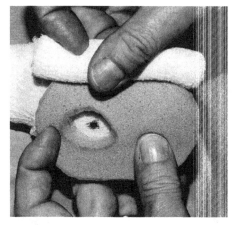

Fig. 4.52. From Effects of bandage configuration on paw pad pressure in dogs: A preliminary study, *Journal of the American Animal Hospital Association*.

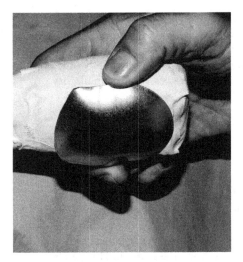

Fig. 4.53.   From Effects of bandage configuration on paw pad pressure in dogs: A preliminary study, *Journal of the American Animal Hospital Association*.

- The final two or three wraps of the secondary layer are done to hold the pad in place.
- For further pressure relief, the paw cup portion of a Mason Metasplint can be placed in the bandage underlying the foam sponge pad (fig. 4.53).
- The tertiary layer of the bandage is applied.

Digital pads

An off-loading foam sponge pad can be used to relieve pressure on the digits of small to medium-sized dogs that have moderate pad wounds, for example, a sutured wound or small open wound, or for orthopedic digital injuries.

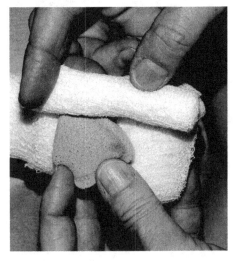

Fig. 4.54.   From Effects of bandage configuration on paw pad pressure in dogs: A preliminary study, *Journal of the American Animal Hospital Association*).

- A piece of medium compressibility (blue color) foam sponge padding (Confor™foam, HiTech Foam, Lincoln, NE) is cut in a triangular shape that is approximately the size of the metacarpal/metatarsal pad. The thickness of the foam pad is split in half with a scalpel blade or razor blade to a thickness of 0.5 inch (1.25 cm).
- The primary and all but the last two or three wraps of the secondary layer of a basic paw and distal limb bandage are applied (see page 56 this chapter, Basic Paw and Distal Limb Bandage).
- The triangular pad is placed on the palmar/plantar surface of the bandage under the metacarpal/metatarsal pad (fig. 4.54).

- The final two or three wraps of the secondary layer are done to hold the pad in place.
- For further pressure relief, the paw cup portion of a Mason Metasplint can be placed in the bandage underlying the foam sponge pad (fig. 4.53).

Aftercare—moderate wounds on small to medium-sized dogs

At the time of bandage change, all parts of the bandage are removed and replaced. The sponge pad, either the donut or triangular shaped, is saved for incorporation in the next bandage. If wound drainage has been absorbed into the pad, it may be necessary to have two pads. Thus, when one pad is soiled by drainage, it can be washed and rinsed with antiseptic solution, be allowed to dry, and be incorporated in the next bandage.

Advantages and complications—moderate wounds on small to medium-sized dogs

The advantage of the foam sponge pad is the pressure relief it provides on any pad wounds that are present. With the donut pad for metacarpal/metatarsal pad off-loading, the principle is that of distributing pressure on tissues around the wound rather than on the wound (fig. 4.55, A). With the triangular pad placed under the metacarpal/metatarsal pad, the off-loading principle is that of elevating the digits by placing padding under the metacarpal/metatarsal pad (fig. 4.55, B). A complication that may be associated with the triangular foam sponge pad is that it may slip out of place as the animal puts weight on the bandage. To help keep the pad in place, a slight concavity can be cut in the side of the pad that goes closest to the metacarpal/metatarsal pad.

Techniques—major reconstructive or salvage paw surgery, especially on large dogs

"Clamshell" splints
"Clamshell" splints can be used for paw pad pressure relief following major paw reconstructive or salvage surgery, such as phalangeal fillet or pad skin graft surgery. Such splints are especially indicated on large dogs.

- A basic paw and distal limb bandage is applied (see page 56 this chapter, Basic Paw and Distal Limb Bandage).
- Additional secondary wrap is applied to the level of the elbow for a forelimb or the hock for the pelvic limb to make the bandage circumferentially equal along its length.

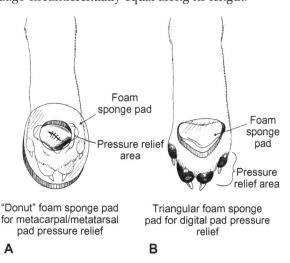

A "Donut" foam sponge pad for metacarpal/metatarsal pad pressure relief

B Triangular foam sponge pad for digital pad pressure relief

Fig. 4.55. Pressure relief on paw pads: (A) Metacarpal/metatarsal pad pressure relief. (B) Digital pad pressure relief.

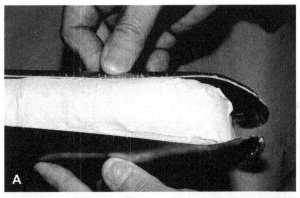

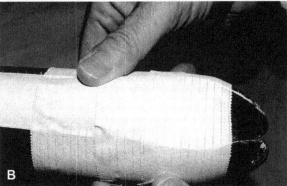

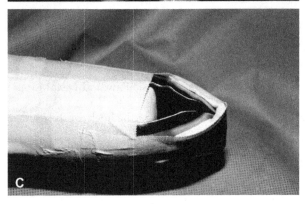

Fig. 4.56.   From *Small Animal Distal Limb Injuries*, published by Teton New Media (in press).

- The tertiary bandage layer of adhesive tape is applied.
- Two metal splints of the appropriate size are placed on opposite sides of the bandage. On the forelimb the splints should extend to near the elbow. On the hind limb they should extend to near the hock. The splints are usually placed on the cranial and volar/plantar bandage surfaces. However, they could be placed on the medial and lateral surfaces. The medial-lateral placement of the splints is primarily indicated on the pelvic limb where splints are placed below the hock. The medial-lateral placement helps avoid the skin irritation that can be caused by the top of the cranial splint as it presses against the skin on the cranial/flexor aspect of the hock. An alternative to medial-lateral splint placement is use of a one-half "clamshell" splint (see One-Half "Clamshell" Splint, below). For a large dog, medial-lateral placement will give more support/stability. The splints are placed with the paw cups facing each other and extending approximately 1 to 1.5 inches (2.5 to 3.8 cm) beyond the paw (fig. 4.56A).
- The splints are taped in place with strips of 2-inch (5.0 cm)-wide adhesive tape (fig. 4.56B). It is important that adhesive tape be used for the tertiary bandage layer and to tape the splints in place. The adhesion of the tape of these two layers between the splints provides security of the splints so they do not slip dorsally with weight bearing.
- Some form of padding, such as two or three gauze sponges, should be taped over the ends of the paw cups to protect them from abrasion and to protect the clients' floors and carpets from damage (fig. 4.56C).

One-half "clamshell" splint

This splint is used to relieve pressure after major paw reconstructive or salvage surgery, such as phalangeal fillet or pad skin graft surgery, on the pelvic limb. A one-half "clamshell" splint prevents irritation to the cranial surface of the hock that can be caused by the proximal end of the cranial part of a full "clamshell" splint when the dog puts weight on the splint.

- The technique for applying the one-half "clamshell" splint is like that for applying a "clamshell" splint. However, the cranial splint is not applied to the hind limb (see "Clamshell" Splints, above).

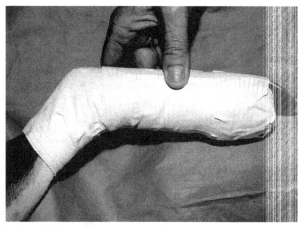

● The length of splint extending beyond the bandage should be shorter than with a "clamshell" splint to provide stability (fig. 4.57).

Fig. 4.57. From *Small Animal Distal Limb Injuries*, published by Teton New Media (in press).

Aftercare—major reconstructive or salvage paw surgery, especially on large dogs

When changing the bandage/splint on a forelimb that has a "clamshell" splint on it, the status of the carpal pad should be noted. If there are signs of pressure injury, the cast padding donut pad should be made thicker to help alleviate pressure on it (see page 58 this chapter, Basic Paw and Distal Limb Bandage, Technique, "Donut" Pads).

When "clamshell" splints are being used on the pelvic limb, the cranial/flexor surface of the tarsal area should be observed for evidence of pressure injury caused by the proximal edge of the cranial splint. If this is noted, the cranial splint can be omitted. If clinical judgment indicates a one-half "clamshell" splint, this can be used. If it is thought that full "clamshell" support is needed, such as for a large dog, then splints can be placed in medial and lateral locations.

Advantages and complications—major reconstructive or salvage paw surgery, especially large dogs

"Clamshell" splints serve as one-limb crutches. They place a limb in a "toe-dancing" position and thus provide maximum relief of pressure on reconstructive and salvage procedures to enhance healing. These splints are especially advantageous for large dogs where their weight could result in significant pressure on repair procedures if it is not reduced or prevented by the splints. The one-half "clamshell" splint has the same advantages as the "clamshell" splint, and it prevents the pressure that can occur on the cranial/flexor tarsal surface.

"Clamshell" splints have the disadvantage of potentially causing pressure injury to the carpal pad if it is not sufficiently padded with a cast padding donut pad. The one-half "clamshell" splint may not provide as much support as a "clamshell" splint.

Dorsal paw pressure relief

Indications

A stockinette padding bandage can be used for temporary padding and coverage of the paws in small dogs and cats. This covering is indicated to prevent abrasive and pressure-type lesions that result from abnormal placement of the paw due to a temporary peripheral nerve lesion that has potential for recovery with time, that is, a neuropraxic nerve lesion (fig. 4.58). Other types of commercial splints and braces are available. However, the author (SFS) has found this bandage to work nicely on small dogs and cats.

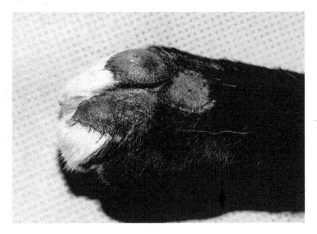

Fig. 4.58.   An example of a dorsal paw pressure/abrasive lesion on which a dorsal paw pressure relief bandage would be indicated. From *Small Animal Distal Limb Injuries*, Teton New Media.

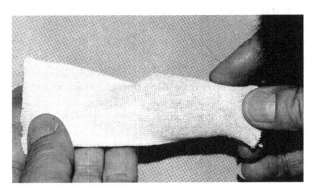

Fig. 4.59.   From *Small Animal Distal Limb Injuries*, published by Teton New Media (in press).

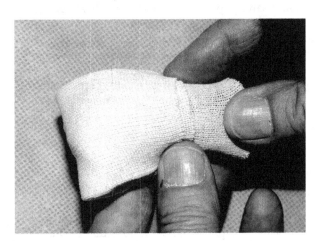

Fig. 4.60.   From *Small Animal Distal Limb Injuries*, published by Teton New Media (in press).

Technique

- A length of 2-inch (5.0 cm)-diameter cotton or synthetic orthopedic stockinette that is used to line casts is placed on the distal limb extending from the proximal metacarpal/metatarsal level to beyond the digits. The stockinette is cut 1 to 2 inches (2.5–5.0 cm) beyond the ends of the digits (fig. 4.59).

- The distal end of the stockinette is folded back onto the paw. The stockinette is folded dorsally if the lesion is on the dorsum of the paw or ventrally if the lesion is on the palmar/plantar paw surface (fig. 4.60).

⦾ A circumferential wrap of 1-inch (2.5cm)-wide adhesive tape is used to tape the distal end of the stockinette in place. The proximal end of the stockinette is also taped in place with a 1-inch (2.5cm)-wide adhesive tape strip that is placed circumferentially with half of its width on the stockinette and half on the haired skin of the limb. This strip may overlap the first strip (fig. 4.61).

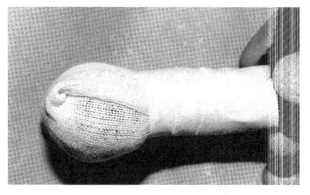

Fig. 4.61. From *Small Animal Distal Limb Injuries*, published by Teton New Media (in press).

Aftercare

⦾ The animal's exercise should be limited and preferably confined to soft surfaces. Keeping the stockinette clean and dry is important.
⦾ Periodically, the stockinette should be observed for signs of wear over the area of the pressure/abrasion lesion to determine if a bandage change is indicated.
⦾ A piece of waterproof tape can be placed over the area of stockinette that receives the most wear to prolong its usefulness and avoid frequent bandage changes.

Advantages and complications

This type of bandage provides three layers of stockinette coverage over the lesion area of small dogs and cats until the animal can position the paw normally following nerve regeneration. This coverage is inexpensive. However, it would not be sufficient for larger dogs due to the wear the animal would place on the stockinette.

Carpal sling

Indications

The carpal sling is indicated to prevent weight-bearing on a forelimb without having to immobilize the entire limb. It is useful for short periods when it is important that the animal not bear weight but when immobility of the entire limb is not required. An orthopedic example is a fracture that has been repaired but is not sufficiently strong to withstand immediate walking forces. A soft tissue example is reconstructive surgery or wound management on a paw pad. The sling allows the elbow and shoulder to flex and extend but prevents the paw from touching the ground.

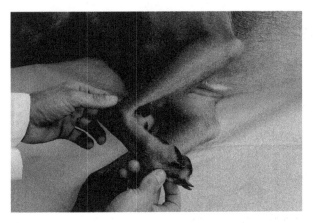

Fig. 4.62.

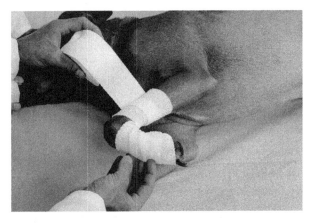

Fig. 4.63.

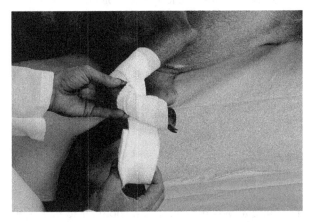

Fig. 4.64.

Technique

- The animal is positioned in lateral recumbency with the affected limb up. The carpus is palpated to assure that flexion is not uncomfortable (fig. 4.62). Many dogs lose mobility in the carpi as they age, and it might be painful if the carpus is flexed for a prolonged period.

- The carpus should be flexed, but not beyond 90 degrees. Excessive flexion may be uncomfortable for the animal. An initial layer of cast padding is applied to the paw and distal antibrachium in a figure-of-eight manner. Excessive bulk around or behind the joint should be avoided. The middle two digits can be left exposed to assess for swelling during aftercare (figs. 4.63, 4.64).

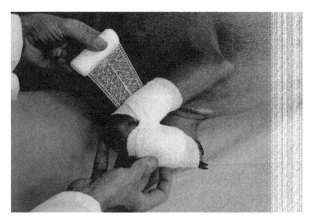

Fig. 4.65.

A second layer of roll gauze is then applied, taking care to avoid tension (fig. 4.65).

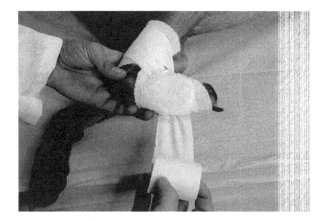

Fig. 4.66.

Finally, 2-inch (5.0 cm)-wide porous adhesive tape is applied in a similar figure-of-eight pattern without tension (fig. 4.66). Using the same type of tape, a final loop is made around the entire bandage (fig. 4.67).

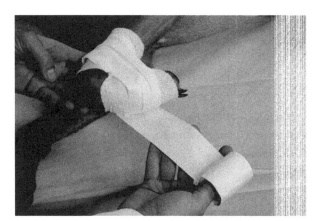

Fig. 4.67.

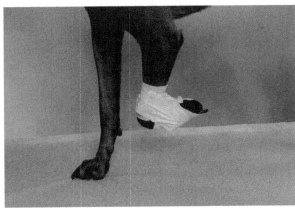

- The animal should then be able to stand comfortably without the sling slipping off (fig. 4.68).

Fig. 4.68.

Aftercare

This animal should be monitored carefully to assure that the toes are not swelling and that the bandage is not slipping. The sling should not be used for longer than two weeks, and it should be checked twice daily during that time.

If the sling is being used as part of the treatment of a paw pad injury, it will be necessary to remove and replace it periodically to allow wound treatment.

Advantages and complications

Movement is important for joint health, and this sling allows motion of the elbow and shoulder joints. This is helpful if an articular fracture of the elbow has been repaired. The sling will result in some temporary stiffness of the carpus after it is removed. Thus, it should not be left in place for longer than two weeks. The biggest complication is that the animal slips the sling off cranially. However, this can be avoided with sufficient carpal flexion and proper application of the figure-of-eight technique.

Basic forelimb splint

This information for splints on the forelimb also applies to the pelvic limb (see page 93 this chapter, Basic Pelvic Limb Splint).

Indications

Splints are used for a variety of purposes, including to support some fractures or ligamentous instability or to protect a surgical repair such as a skin graft over a joint.

Technique

Although pictures for this technique are for a forelimb splint, the principles of the technique are the same for applying a splint to the pelvic limb. Splints may be purchased from various companies or may be fashioned in a custom manner using fiberglass tape or temperature-dependent plastics.

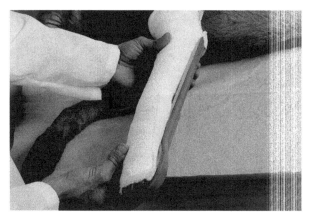

Fig. 4.69.

- The initial steps in application of a splint are the same as for applying a soft padded bandage (see page 47 this chapter, Forelimb Bandages, Casts, and Splints; Basic Soft Padded Limb Bandage). The steps are followed up through the application of the roll gauze. The final protective layer is not applied.
- After applying the roll gauze, an appropriate splint is selected. If a commercial product is used, whether plastic or aluminum, assure that it fits well with the size of the animal and amount of padding that has been used (figs. 4.69, 4.70). The length of the splint may be trimmed if necessary.
- The splint should then be secured to the limb using roll gauze (figs. 4.71, 4.72). The gauze should not be a stretchable variety and should be applied firmly but without tension.

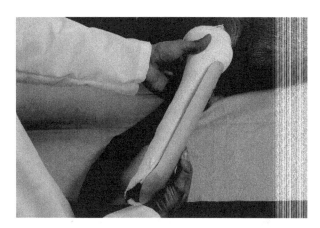

Fig. 4.70.

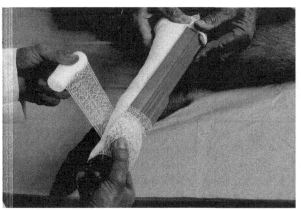

Fig. 4.71.

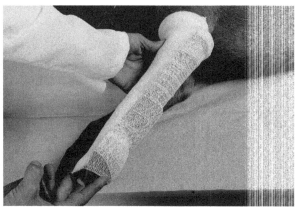

Fig. 4.72.

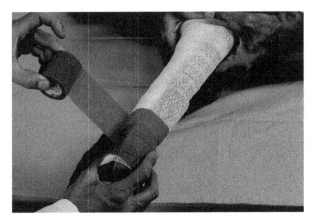

Fig. 4.73.

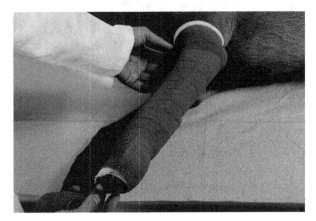

Fig. 4.74.

- A final protective layer (2 inch [5.0 cm] wide porous adhesive tape or elastic adhesive tape) should then be added (figs. 4.73, 4.74).
- If fiberglass casting tape is used, the initial steps are the same. The width of the casting tape chosen should be sufficient to cover at least one-third of the circumference of the limb. The casting tape may either be wetted as a roll and then unrolled on the limb or unrolled on a flat surface prior to being wetted. In either case, it is vital to avoid stretching the casting tape when it is being unrolled as it will slowly shrink back which may excessively shorten the splint. The warmer the water is to wet the tape, the quicker it will harden. Beginners should use colder water to wet the tape. It is best to use gloved hands while handling the fiberglass so that the resin on the tape does not stick to the user's skin.

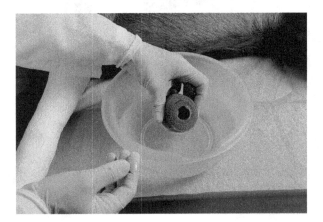

Fig. 4.75.

- If casting tape is wetted while it is rolled, the water should be worked all the way through the roll prior to forming the splint. Placing the roll in the water and lifting it out in a scooping-type motion so the edge of the tape is facing up may allow water to be pulled down through the tape by gravity. After the roll is thoroughly wetted, excess water should be squeezed out so the underlying bandage does not absorb the moisture (figs. 4.75, 4.76).

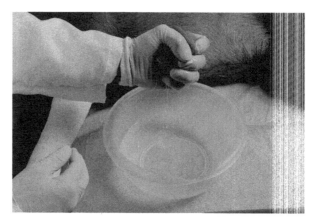

Fig. 4.76.

• The end of the tape is held at one end of the limb, and it is unrolled up and down the length of the bandage several times to layer the tape on the bandage. The layering should continue until sufficient thickness is achieved, at which point the tape is cut (fig. 4.77).

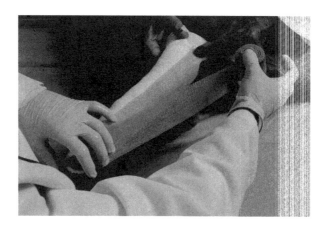

Fig. 4.77.

• The tape is then carefully smoothed and shaped to conform to the limb (fig. 4.78). The splint is then secured to the limb using roll gauze before it sets (figs. 4.79, 4.80). It is important that all the layers of the fiberglass bond to each other. Thus, movement of the patient or splint should be avoided while the fiberglass is hardening. Furthermore, pressure on the hardening splint with fingers or by table edges should be avoided because indentations may result in pressure sores.

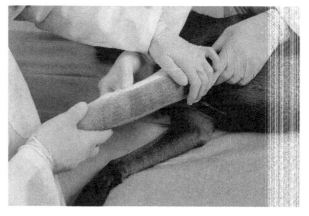

Fig. 4.78.

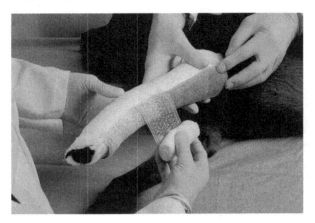

Fig. 4.79.

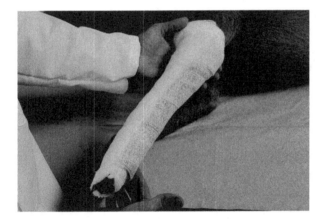

Fig. 4.80.

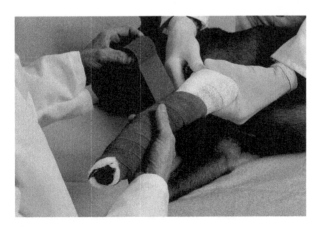

Fig. 4.81.

- When the splint has hardened, an outer protective layer of 2 inch (5.0 cm) wide porous adhesive tape or elastic adhesive tape is added (fig. 4.81).

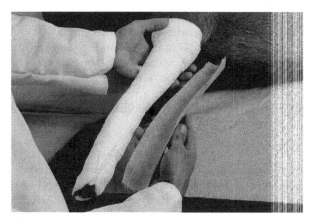

Fig. 4.82.

- If the bandage needs to be changed, the splint may be reused if it is in good condition (fig. 4.82).

Aftercare

The bandage and splint should be carefully monitored. They should be kept clean and dry, and the animal should not be allowed to lick or chew at them. The two exposed digits should be examined for signs of swelling (separation of the digits), which would indicate the bandage is too tight and needs to be changed. A veterinarian should be contacted if the animal's use of the limb decreases.

If the bandage and splint have been used to treat a draining wound, periodic bandage change will be necessary (see page 47 this chapter, Forelimb Bandages, Casts, and Splints; Basic Soft Padded Limb Bandage).

Advantages and complications

The soft padded bandage portion of the appliance is easy to apply, and it provides some support and protection for a variety of conditions. The addition of a splint provides an additional moderate amount of stability, and it is easy to place and remove. The bandage and splint combination are a good means of immobilizing joints when wound management requires such immobility. General complications include bandage and splint slipping, pressure wounds, and mutilation by the animal. If any of these are suspected, the bandage and splint should be changed. Each area of the bandage has its advantages and complications (see page 47 this chapter, Forelimb Bandages, Casts, and Splints; Basic Soft Padded Limb Bandage).

Basic forelimb cast

The information for casts on the pelvic limb also applies to the forelimb (see page 93 this chapter, Pelvic Limb Bandages, Casts, and Splints; Basic Pelvic Limb Cast).

Spica bandage and lateral splint

Indications

The spica bandage and splint is a method of immobilizing the entire forelimb in extension. This bandage and splint can be used when moderate immobilization of the forelimb area is required. It is particularly useful for upper limb immobilization. Some indications include scapular fractures or to support surgical stabilization of elbow luxations. Additionally, the spica bandage and splint is indicated for conservative treatment of lateral shoulder luxations or to provide support following surgical repair. It is not recommended to manage medial shoulder luxations.

For soft tissue injuries, the spica bandage and splint are primarily indicated for managing wounds over the point of the elbow, such as elbow hygromas and open or closed wounds over the olecranon. Healing of wounds in this location require *extension* and *immobilization*, which the spica bandage and splint provide. Extension keeps the animal from bending the elbow to get in sternal recumbency which would put pressure on the area. Immobilization keeps the tissues from moving so they can heal.

Technique

The spica bandage and splint utilizes standard bandage material and incorporates either fiberglass casting material or aluminum splint rod. The bandage and splint can be applied with the animal standing or in lateral recumbency with the affected limb up. Application is generally easier with the animal standing, but that requires some degree of cooperation from the animal. If the animal is in lateral recumbency, it must be frequently lifted in order to pass the bandage material around the thorax. When an animal is anesthetized, care must be taken to avoid excessive tightness, which might interfere with chest excursions and respiration.

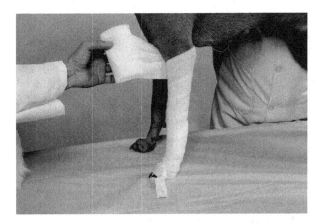

Fig. 4.83.

- Application of a spica bandage and splint begins with several layers of cast padding. The bandage should begin at the digits and progress up the limb as would be the case for an ordinary soft padded bandage (fig. 4.83).

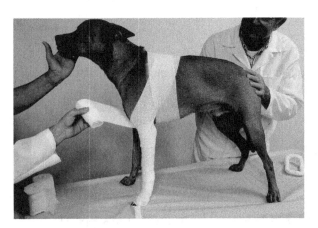

Fig. 4.84.

- The cast padding is then continued over the dorsum of the animal and around the thorax both in front and behind the limb (figs. 4.84, 4.85).

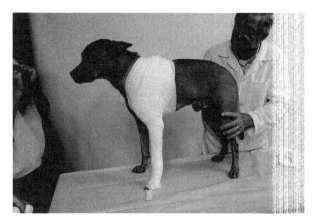

Fig. 4.85.

Care should be taken with all layers to avoid wrapping the bandage too tightly around the thorax. After two to three layers of cast padding are applied, a layer of roll gauze is unrolled over the padding to secure the bandage (fig. 4.86).

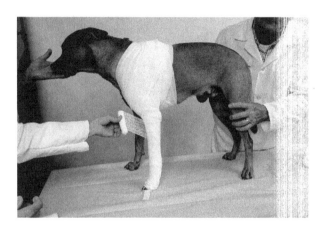

Fig. 4.86.

Fiberglass casting tape is the best material to use for the splint. It may be unrolled to the proper length to extend from the digits to over the shoulder area prior to its wetting, or it may be wetted and unrolled on the patient as shown (fig. 4.87). Alternatively, a length of aluminum splint rod can be bent in the shape of an elongated loop that extends from the digits to over the shoulders. It is then fashioned to the curvatures of the lateral aspect of the limb as much as possible.

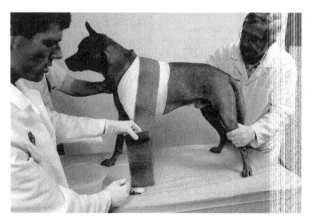

Fig. 4.87.

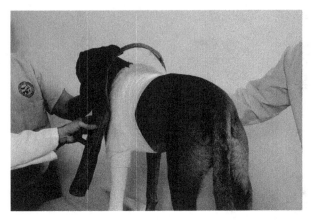

Fig. 4.88.

- The casting tape must extend over the dorsum and down the opposite side of the thorax slightly in order to properly immobilize the limb (fig. 4.88).

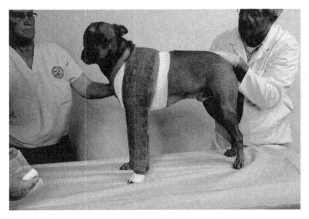

Fig. 4.89.

- The casting tape should be fashioned in a broad enough manner to cover the lateral aspect of the shoulder area and extend slightly around the cranial portion of the shoulder joint (fig. 4.89).

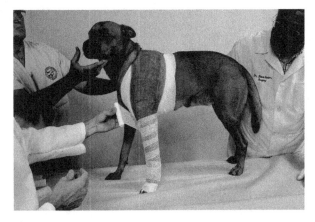

Fig. 4.90.

- The casting material or aluminum splint rod loop is then held in place with an additional layer of roll gauze. If casting material is used, it is allowed to dry (figs. 4.90, 4.91). It is important that the animal not be allowed to move during the drying of the splint if fiberglass casting material has been used.

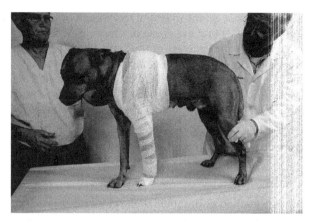

Fig. 4.91.

- Finally, a protective outer layer is wrapped over the splint, avoiding undue tension (fig. 4.92).
- If the splint has been applied as part of the treatment of a wound over the point of the elbow, a window can be cut in the splint and bandage over this area to allow wound care.

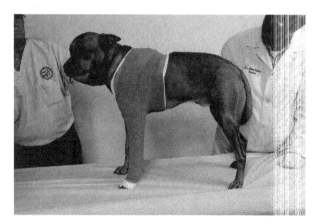

Fig. 4.92.

Aftercare

The bandage and splint should be monitored closely. Observation is important to be sure the animal is not having trouble breathing and that there is no slippage of the bandage and splint or limb underneath. If the limb seems to have excessive motion, the front of the shoulder may be slipping out of the cranial aspect of the splint.

For wound care over the point of the elbow, treatment is done through the window in the splint and bandage. A small bandage is placed over the window following each treatment. If lavage is done on the wound, measures should be taken to avoid getting the bandage material around the window wet.

Advantages and complications

The spica bandage and splint provides a good method for immobilizing the entire forelimb. It does not provide rigid support, so it is not sufficient to immobilize most fractures below the scapula. If an aluminum splint rod loop is used for the lateral splint, it may not immobilize the front of the shoulder as well and may not be as comfortable for the animal.

Because of its length and immobility, the splint is somewhat awkward for the animal. Most animals will adapt after a few days, but some will not tolerate it. Special care should be taken to assure that the animal does not get into a lateral recumbent position from which it is unable to rise. This may be especially true for animals that are obese or otherwise debilitated.

When the splint is used to treat soft tissue wounds over the point of the elbow, it provides the immobilization and extension necessary for soft tissue healing. When a window is cut over the point of the elbow, it conserves on bandage materials since only the portion of bandage over the wound is changed daily. If the portion of the bandage around the window becomes wet during wound care, it can become a source of bacterial growth. Thus, care must be used in cleaning the wound surface.

Aluminum rod loop elbow splint

Indications

Another method to immobilize the elbow is to use a cranially-applied splint made from aluminum splint rod. The splint is primarily indicated to provide immobilization and extension of the elbow to support the healing of soft tissue wounds over the point of the elbow, such as elbow hygromas and open or closed wounds over the olecranon. The splint does not immobilize the shoulder at all.

Technique

The splint can be applied with the patient standing or in lateral recumbency with the affected limb up. The choice of position may depend on the animal's body shape.

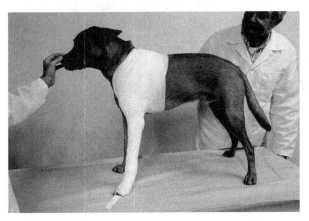

Fig. 4.93.

- If an open or closed wound is present in the area, the appropriate medication and primary bandage layer are applied to the wound.
- A soft-padded bandage secondary layer is wrapped around the elbow area. On animals with long, thin legs, the bandage is extended into the axilla and stopped. On other animals, it may be necessary to continue this wrap over the shoulders and around the thorax in the form of a spica bandage (fig. 4.93; see page 83 this chapter, Spica Bandage and Lateral Splint).

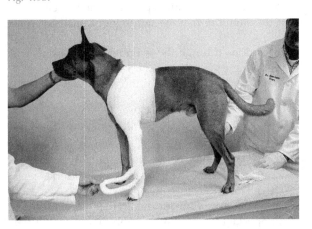

Fig. 4.94.

- A section of the appropriate-sized aluminum splint rod is bent into a narrow rectangle, and an angle is bent at the midpoint of the long sides of the rectangle (fig. 4.94).

- The splint should conform to the natural standing angle of the elbow and fit closely against the bandage with the bend of the splint positioned at the bend of the elbow (fig. 4.95). The splint is then secured using roll gauze and an outer protective layer.
- If a wound is to be treated over the point of the elbow, a window can be cut in the bandage over the wound to allow treatment.

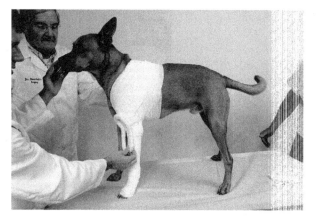

Fig. 4.95.

Aftercare

The bandage and splint should be monitored carefully. The animal should be closely observed to note any change in its willingness to put weight on the leg, as this could indicate slippage or formation of a bandage sore. In this case, the bandage and splint should be changed.

If a wound is being treated over the point of the elbow, treatment is done through the window in the bandage. A small bandage is placed over the window following each treatment. If lavage is done on the wound, measures should be taken to avoid getting the bandage material around the window wet.

Advantages and complications

This bandage and splint are easier to apply and may be better tolerated than a spica bandage and splint since the shoulder is not immobilized. It provides the immobilization and extension necessary for soft tissue healing. When a window is cut over the point of the elbow, it conserves on bandage material since only a portion of bandage over the wound is changed daily. If the portion of the bandage around the window becomes wet during wound care, it can become a source of bacterial growth. Thus, care should be used in cleaning the wound surface.

Velpeau sling

Indications

The Velpeau sling can be used to prevent weight bearing on a forelimb in a variety of situations. If the only purpose is to prevent weight bearing, such as following placement of pad grafts, a carpal sling may be more comfortable than a Velpeau sling since the latter places both the carpus and elbow in tight flexion (see page 75 this chapter, Carpal Sling).

The Velpeau sling also helps to lateralize the proximal humerus and is therefore useful in conservative management of medial shoulder luxations. This lateralizing effect makes it unsuitable for lateral shoulder luxations and for some scapular fractures.

Technique

The Velpeau sling supports the front limb in a flexed position against the animal's thorax (fig. 4.96). The sling is applied using standard layers of material in order to pad, support, and protect. The sling can be applied with the animal standing or in lateral recumbency with the affected limb up. Application is generally easier with the animal standing, but it requires some degree of cooperation from the patient.

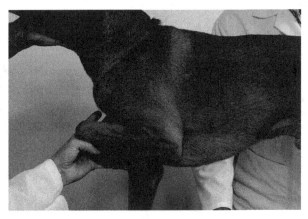

Fig. 4.96.   Front limb is being held in the position that the Velpeau sling will ultimately maintain.

When the animal is in lateral recumbency, it must be lifted frequently to pass the bandage material around the thorax. When an animal is anesthetized, care must be taken to avoid excessive tightness, which might interfere with chest excursions and respiration.

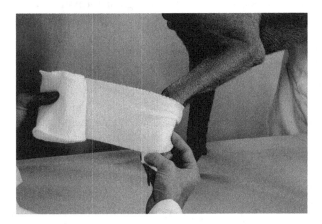

Fig. 4.97.

- The Velpeau sling application is begun by using cast padding to wrap around the limb distal to the carpus, wrapping two to three times (fig. 4.97).

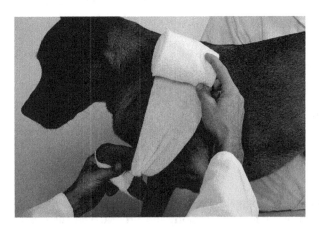

Fig. 4.98.

- While holding the limb in the desired flexed position, the cast padding is brought up over the dorsum of the animal and around the thorax back to the limb to hold it in the flexed position against the thorax (fig. 4.98).

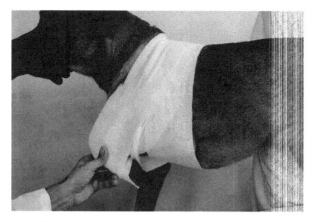

Fig. 4.99.

- The cast padding wrapping is continued until two to three layers have covered the thorax and flexed limb, to include the front of the carpus (fig. 4.99).

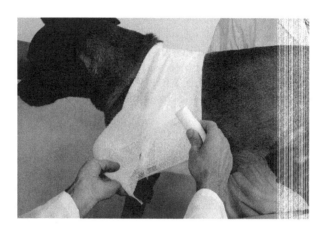

Fig. 4.100.

- A similar wrapping pattern is placed over this initial layer using roll gauze or white tape (fig. 4.100).

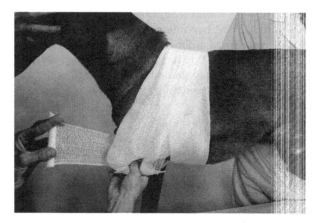

Fig. 4.101.

- Care should be taken to ensure that the wrapping material supports the front of the carpus so the limb cannot slip cranially out of the sling (fig. 4.101).

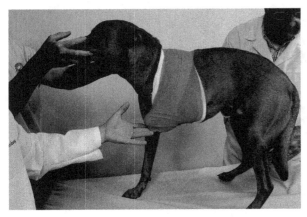

● Finally, a protective outer layer of 2 inch (5.0 cm) wide porous adhesive tape or elastic adhesive tape is applied to the sling (fig. 4.102).

Fig. 4.102.

Aftercare

The sling should be closely monitored. Vigilance is important to be sure the animal is not having any trouble breathing and that there is no slippage of the sling or limb underneath. The sling should be left in place only as long as necessary to treat the primary problem. However, its presence beyond two weeks may result in problems. After removing the sling, activity should be gradually increased over several weeks to allow the tissues to adjust to restoration of mobility.

Advantages and complications

The Velpeau sling provides a secure method of immobilizing the forelimb. However, it is confining and may be slightly uncomfortable for the animal initially. If it is applied too tightly, movement of the chest wall could be compromised, causing respiratory distress. If the flexed carpus and paw are compressed by elastic gauze or tape, if the sling loosens or slips, or if there is preexisting vascular obstruction of the paw, there may be necrosis of the skin and underlying structures. Because all joints of the limb are immobilized, cartilage health is compromised, and lameness may be present when the sling is removed. If the sling is used more than two weeks, joint contracture can occur due to the severe flexion of the forelimb joints.

When attempting to immobilize the axillary area of a cat to support the healing of a wound in this area, a Velpeau sling would seem to be indicated in principle; however, this sling is not tolerated well by cats. One author (SFS) has found that immobilization of the axillary region on a cat is best accomplished by cage rest and a cardboard box. A box large enough to accommodate the cat is placed up-side-down in the cat's cage. The box has a hole cut in its side that is large enough for the cat to get through. Cats like to get in such accommodations and will sit in sternal recumbency in the box with all limbs flexed, thus gaining some immobilization of the axillary region. A large opened paper sack will also serve this purpose.

Pelvic limb bandages, casts, and splints

Basic soft padded limb bandage

The information for the basic soft padded limb bandage on the forelimb also applies to the pelvic limb (see page 47 this chapter, Forelimb Bandages, Casts, and Splints; Basic Soft Padded Limb Bandage).

Basic pelvic limb splint

The information for splints on the forelimb also applies to the pelvic limb (see page 78 this chapter, Basic Forelimb Splint).

Basic pelvic limb cast

The information for casts on the pelvic limb also applies to the forelimb (see page 83 this chapter, Basic Forelimb Cast).

Indications

Casting can be performed to address a variety of situations in which immobilization of a portion of a limb is needed. Although a cast does not provide rigid stabilization of bones, the support is often sufficient to allow healing of selected fractures. Additionally, casts can be used to provide support postoperatively in cases such as arthrodeses or soft tissue reconstructions. If necessary, casts can be split longitudinally into two halves ("bivalving") and be reapplied. This would be indicated if the cast were being used for immobilization of a wound that needed periodic treatment or to check for and accommodate limb swelling (see Advantages and Complications, below). Half of the splint cast can be used as a splint. However, this decreases the stability compared to a cast.

Technique

Although the pictures for this technique are for a pelvic limb cast, the principles of the technique are the same for applying a cast to a forelimb.

- The initial steps in application of a cast are similar to those for a soft padded bandage. However, there are some important differences. Tape "stirrups" are placed and cotton pieces are placed in the interdigital and interpad areas as with a soft padded bandage (see page 47 this chapter, Forelimb Bandages and Splints, Basic Soft Padded Bandage).
- Regular cast: Throughout cast application, the limb should be held in a neutral position with each joint moderately flexed in a functional manner.
- A length of stockinette is cut to twice the length of the limb to be casted. The length used to measure should extend proximal to the most proximal extent of the proposed cast by two to three inches (5.0–7.6 cm) and beyond the digits by a similar distance (fig. 4.103).

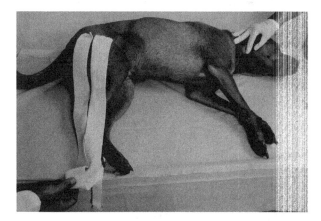

Fig. 4.103.

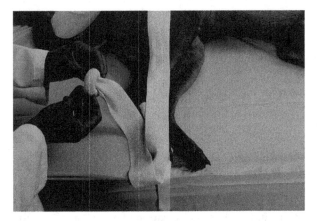

Fig. 4.104.

- The stockinette is doubled onto itself to create a double thickness, and it is placed on the limb. The author (WCR) finds it easiest to do this by rolling half the length of the stockinette from one end in a conventional manner (fig. 4.104) and rolling from the opposite end by rolling the stockinette in on itself (fig. 4.105).

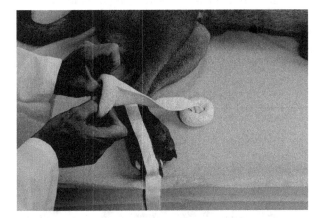

Fig. 4.105.

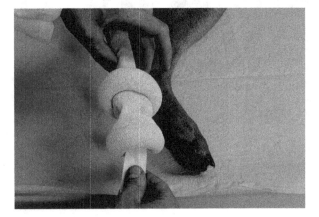

Fig. 4.106.

- The end of the stockinette that was rolled conventionally is then rolled up onto the limb. The remaining portion is then easily unrolled over the first layer (figs. 4.106, 4.107, 4.108). It is important to leave several inches of stockinette protruding beyond the end of the digits.
- "Donuts" of padding are placed over bony prominences as described for soft padded bandages. These donuts are usually placed under the stockinette. Thus, the stockinette holds them in place. It is important that they do not slip out of place as the remaining bandage layers are applied.

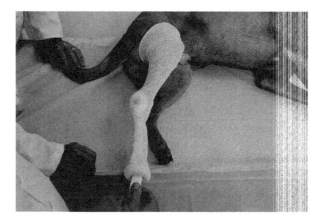

Fig. 4.107.

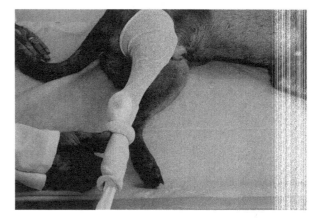

Fig. 4.108.

● Cast padding (fig. 4.109) and then roll gauze (fig. 4.110) are placed over the stockinette as described for a soft padded bandage. Generally, about three to four plies of cast padding are sufficient (It should be remembered that by overlapping fifty percent, each "layer" of bandage material actually adds two thicknesses of material). The stockinette should protrude from each end of the bandage (fig. 4.111).

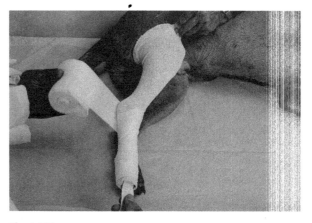

Fig. 4.109.

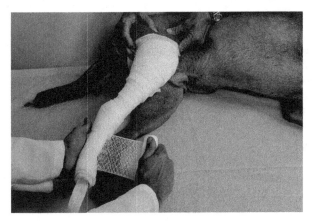

Fig. 4.110.

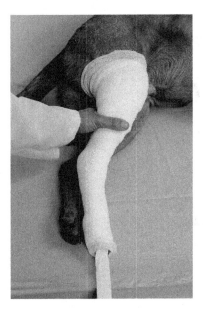

Fig. 4.111.

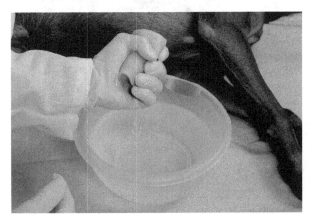

Fig. 4.112.

 Examination gloves should be donned and the fiberglass casting material to be used should be thoroughly wetted. Warm water will result in the cast's setting more quickly. Thus, beginners should use colder water to allow more time for application. It is important to work the water all the way to the innermost layers of the roll. Placing the roll in the water and lifting it out in a scooping motion so the edge of the tape is facing up may allow water to be pulled down through the tape by gravity. After it is completely saturated, the roll should be squeezed to eliminate excess water so the underlying bandage does not absorb the moisture (fig. 4.112).

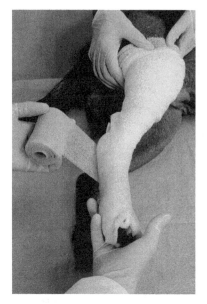

- The casting tape is applied from distal to proximal being careful to achieve fifty percent overlap with each wrap and to avoid wrinkles (fig. 4.113). Care should be taken not to place tension on the tape as it is applied since that will result in the cast's becoming excessively tight.

Fig. 4.113.

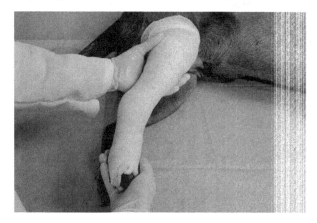

- The distal end of the casting tape layer should be even with the end of the digits, with the underlying layers extending past the fiberglass by 1 to 2 inches (2.5–5.0 cm).
- Additional rolls of casting tape are applied until the desired thickness is achieved. The final result should be a smooth cast with each layer bonded to those beneath (fig. 4.114).

Fig. 4.114.

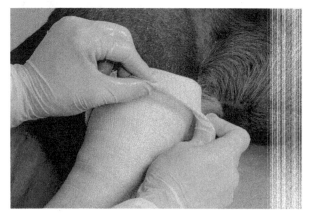

- Before the cast hardens, the stockinette and cast padding are pulled over each end of the cast to create a padded edge over the ends of the cast (fig. 4.115).

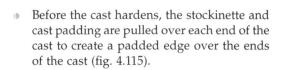

Fig. 4.115.

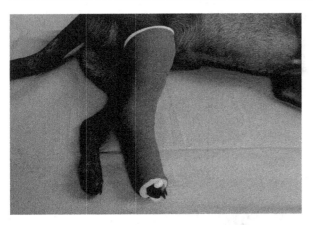

Fig. 4.116.

- The cast is allowed to harden. During hardening, care should be taken not to allow fingers or rigid supports (table edges, etc.) to indent the cast as this could predispose to pressure wounds.
- The "stirrups" are folded up against the distal end of the cast. A final protective layer of 2 inch (5.0 cm) wide porous adhesive tape or elastic adhesive tape is applied after the cast has hardened (fig. 4.116).

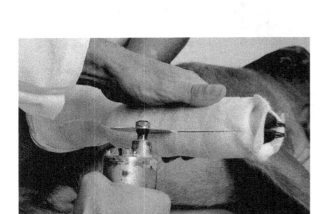

Fig. 4.117.

- "Bivalving" a cast: A cast cutting saw can be used to make a bivalved cast that can be removed and replaced periodically. A cast-cutting saw is used to split the cast longitudinally along the lateral and medial aspects for the forelimb or the cranial and caudal aspects for the pelvic limb (fig. 4.117). Cast splitters are helpful to separate the two halves of the cast (figs. 4.118, 4.119). At times the two halves of the cast can be reapplied (fig. 4.120).

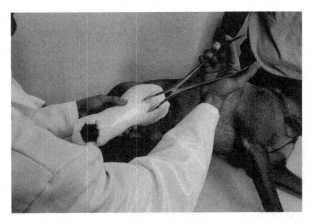

Fig. 4.118.

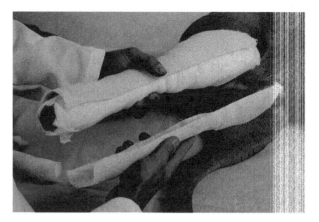

Fig. 4.119.

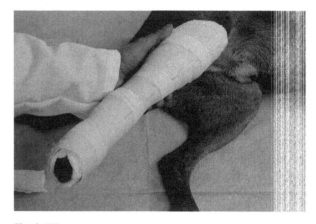

Fig. 4.120.

Aftercare

The cast should be carefully monitored. It should be kept clean and dry, and the animal should not be allowed to lick or chew at it. The two exposed digits should be examined for signs of swelling (separation of the digits), which would indicate the cast is too tight and needs to be changed or bivalved. A veterinarian should be contacted if the animal's use of the limb decreases.

If the cast has been used to immobilize a draining wound, periodic bandage change will be necessary. Thus, a bivalved cast will be necessary to allow periodic removal for bandage change (see page 47 this chapter, Forelimb Bandages, Casts, and Splints; Basic Soft Padded Limb Bandage). Alternatively, one-half of the cast can be applied to the limb as a splint, with the application on the side opposite the location of the wound.

Advantages and complications

A cast provides the most rigid stabilization of a limb. Because it is so rigid, and because it may be in place for a longer period, casts can result in pressure wounds, especially over bony prominences. Early detection is the key to preventing serious problems. If there is any indication that a problem is developing (i.e., wet or dirty cast, spots on the cast, offensive odor to the cast, decreased limb use, or licking and chewing at the cast), the cast should be removed and the limb should be inspected. If necessary, the two halves of the cast may be replaced after new inner bandage layers are applied. Pressure wounds that do develop should be cared for and adjustments should be made to prevent further pressure by the cast, such as not applying the cast directly over the wound. For example, when using the cast that has been split for removal, one-half of the cast can be used as a splint on the opposite side of the limb, or cutting a window in the cast over the wound can be considered.

Early placement of a cast on a limb where there has been trauma resulting in fractures with no displacement can have the potential for complications. With the cast in place, there is no accommodation for the edema that will result over the first few days following injury. Thus, the swelling of the limb that is confined in the cast may encroach on blood vessels. The result can be ischemic necrosis of soft tissues. In such cases, a bivalved cast should be considered until swelling subsides.

Ehmer sling

Indications

The Ehmer sling is used to maintain the head of the femur in the acetabulum following closed reduction of a cranio-dorsal coxofemoral luxation. It should not be used to support reduction after a ventral luxation.

Prior to placing an Ehmer sling, it is important to assure that proper case selection has occurred in order to maximize the chances of success. Animals with chronic luxation, poor conformation, avulsions within the joint, or other injuries are usually poor candidates for closed reduction of coxofemoral luxation. Additionally, appropriate technique in reducing the joint is vital.

Technique

This sling should provide internal rotation of the limb, flexion of the hip, and abduction of the limb. The sling is usually placed with the animal in lateral recumbency with the affected limb up. The limb should be held flexed with slight internal rotation of the lower limb.

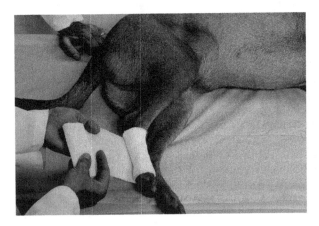

- An initial two to three layers of cast padding are placed around the metatarsal area to begin the application (fig. 4.121).

Fig. 4.121.

● Two-inch (5.0 cm)-wide porous adhesive tape is used for the remainder of the bandage. The tape is initially placed on the metatarsal area by placing it around the caudal surface with the adhesive side of the tape against the initial wrap. The tape is brought cranially in such a way that the adhesive sides meet cranially (fig. 4.122). Thus, the tape does not completely encircle the metatarsal area. This technique helps to guard against placing tape too tightly around the metatarsal area.

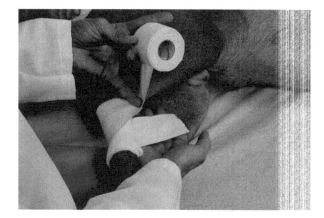

Fig. 4.122.

● The tape is then brought, adhesive side against the animal, up the medial aspect of the crus and around the cranial aspect of the thigh just proximal to the stifle (fig. 4.123).

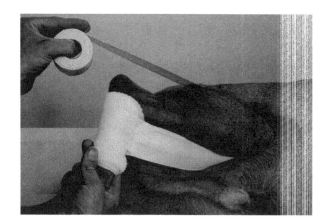

Fig. 4.123.

● The tape then continues around the caudal aspect of the crus and onto the medial side of the hock to then finish caudally on the metatarsal area (figs. 4.124, 4.125). This layer can be repeated. When this portion of the bandage is completed, the lateral aspect of the crus should be visible (i.e., no tape should have crossed the lateral aspect of the hock). Internal rotation should be maintained.

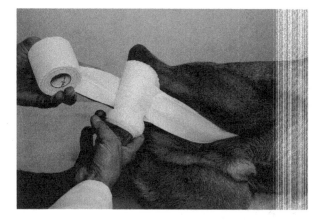

Fig. 4.124.

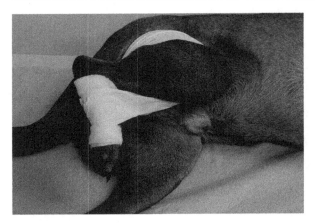

Fig. 4.125.

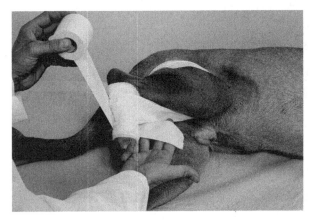

Fig. 4.126.

• The abdominal support portion of the sling begins with tape being applied at the metatarsal region as previously described (fig. 4.126).

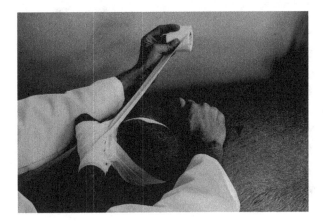

Fig. 4.127.

• The tape is brought up the lateral aspect of the limb and then over the dorsum of the animal. In order to avoid a shift in the skin, which would let the limb slip down as soon as the animal stands, the skin of the flank should gently be pulled ventrally (arrow) before the tape is applied (fig. 4.127).

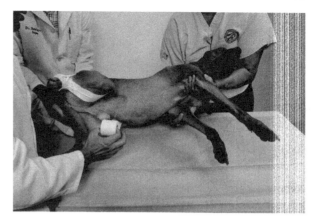

Fig. 4.128.

The tape is continued around the opposite side of the animal and around the ventral aspect of the animal (fig. 4.128). Care is taken to bring the tape cranial to the prepuce on male dogs (fig. 4.129).

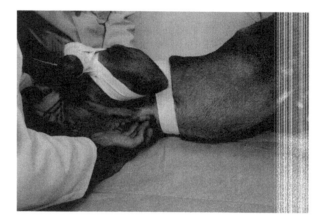

Fig. 4.129.

The layer may be repeated. When completed, the limb should be abducted and flexed, with slight internal rotation (figs. 4.130, 4.131).

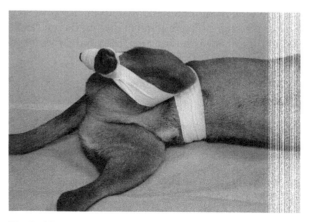

Fig. 4.130.

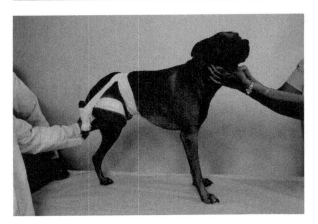

Fig. 4.131.

Aftercare

The Ehmer sling has a higher likelihood of causing bandage-related wounds than some other bandages because the skin is thin where it is applied and because tape is applied directly to the skin. Special care should be taken to watch for slipping of the sling and the development of bandage-related wounds. One particular area to be observed for a pressure wound is the caudal aspect of the metatarsal area. If any wounds develop, the sling should be modified immediately or removed.

Recheck visits with the veterinarian are advised, and the sling should not be left in place for more than 10 to 14 days. Removal of the sling can be uncomfortable for an animal since the tape has been applied directly to the skin. Commercial products are available to help remove adhesive tape bandages. Following removal, the animal should be confined for an additional two to four weeks while it regains range of motion in the limb.

Upon having the Ehmer sling removed, an animal may not use the limb for a day or two because of stiffness. The animal should not be forced to use the limb; however, it should be assured that the coxo-femoral joint is still in place. The animal should improve consistently with each day.

Advantages and complications

The Ehmer sling accomplishes the necessary positioning of the pelvic limb that counters the tendency for relaxation following cranio-dorsal hip luxation. Such positioning would be contraindicated for luxations in other directions. Bandage-related wounds can result from an Ehmer sling, so careful attention must be paid to the calcaneal tendon area, the caudal metatarsal area, the inguinal area, and the medial thigh and crus areas.

90/90 sling

Indications

The 90/90 sling is a method for preventing weight-bearing on a pelvic limb and/or achieving flexion of the hock and stifle joints. Thus, it would be indicated for treating orthopedic conditions where these qualities are needed. It could be considered for preventing weight-bearing on a paw where significant surgery had been done on the pads, such as pad grafts.

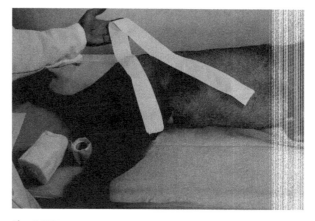

Fig. 4.132.

Technique

- The animal is placed in lateral recumbency with the affected limb up.
- A length of 2-inch (5.0 cm)-wide porous adhesive tape is reserved for later use (fig. 4.132).

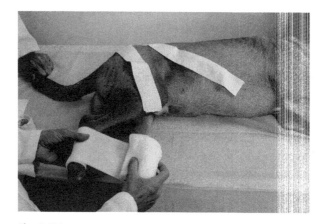

Fig. 4.133.

- An initial cover of two to three layers of cast padding are wrapped around the metatarsals to begin the bandage (fig. 4.133).

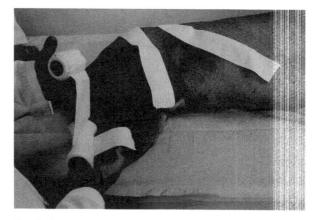

Fig. 4.134.

- Two-inch (5.0 cm)-wide porous adhesive tape is used for the remainder of the bandage. The tape is initially placed on the metatarsal area by placing it around the caudal surface with the adhesive side against the initial wrap. The tape is brought cranially in such a way that the adhesive sides meet cranially (figs. 4.134, 4.135). Thus, the tape does not completely encircle the metatarsal area. This technique helps to guard against placing tape too tightly around the metatarsal area.

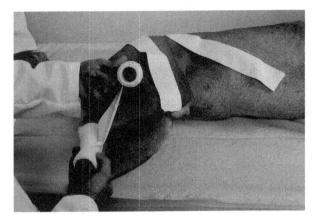

Fig. 4.135.

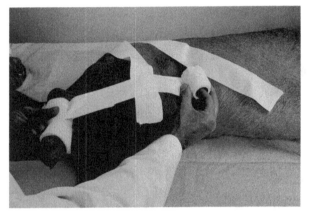

Fig. 4.136.

- The reserved piece of tape (see above) is laid adhesive side up along the femoral area.
- With the hock and stifle flexed, the tape that began on the metatarsal area is brought up the lateral aspect of the crus and around the cranial aspect of the femoral area, with the adhesive side against the animal (fig. 4.136). This tape should cross over the reserved piece of tape at a 90-degree angle. The reserved piece should extend 4 to 6 inches (10–15.2 cm) ventrally past the crossing piece.

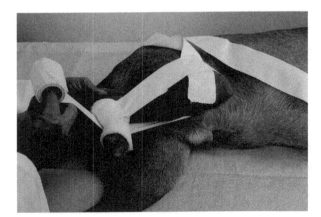

Fig. 4.137.

- The tape that started on the metatarsal area is then brought down the medial aspect of the crus and returned around the caudal aspect of the hock (fig. 4.137). This layer is repeated.

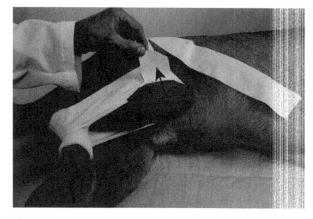

Fig. 4.138.

- The ventral end of the reserved piece of tape is now folded over to secure its attachment to the tape that started on the metatarsal area (fig. 4.138).

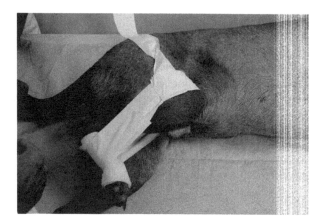

Fig. 4.139.

- The remaining portion of this tape is now twisted to be adhesive side against the patient. It is brought up the femoral area for passage around the dorsum of the animal (fig. 4.139).

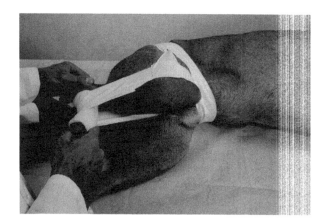

Fig. 4.140.

- It is then brought down the other side and around the abdomen in a manner similar to that illustrated for the Ehmer sling.
- In a male dog, care is taken to assure that the tape does not interfere with the prepuce (fig. 4.140).

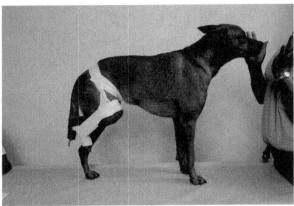

Fig. 4.141.

• The final sling should maintain flexion of the hock and stifle when the animal stands (fig. 4.141).

Aftercare

The 90/90 sling has a higher likelihood of causing bandage-related wounds than some other bandages because the skin is thin where it is applied and because tape is applied directly to the skin. Special care should be taken to watch for slipping of the sling and development of bandage-related wounds. One particular area to be observed for a pressure wound is the caudal aspect of the metatarsal area. If any wounds develop, the sling should be modified immediately or removed.

Recheck visits with the veterinarian are advised, and the sling should not be left in place for more than 10 to 14 days. Removal of the sling can be uncomfortable for an animal since the tape has been applied directly to the skin. Commercial products are available to help remove adhesive tape bandages.

Upon removal of the sling, an animal may not use the limb for a day or two because of stiffness. Limb use will gradually increase with time.

Advantages and complications

The 90/90 sling is less complicated and more comfortable than an Ehmer sling. It serves as a good means to limit weight-bearing on a hind limb and will maintain flexion of most joints in the leg. It does not allow range of motion exercises and may be prone to cause bandage-related wounds.

Tie-over bandage

Indications

The tie-over bandage can be used to protect open, sutured, or grafted wounds on the proximal aspect of the pelvic limb. The bandage can also be used for wounds in the pelvic area.

Technique

See page 29 in chapter 3, Thoracic, Abdominal Tie-Over Bandage.

Aftercare

See page 29 in chapter 3, Thoracic, Abdominal Tie-Over Bandage.

Advantages and complications

The main advantage of a tie-over bandage is that it is an economical form of bandage. The large amounts of secondary and tertiary bandage material that would be required for a circumferential bandage of a proximal limb or truncal bandage are not necessary for a tie-over bandage. The centripetal force from tying the umbilical tape or elastic strip can be considered as a supplement to wound contraction when treating an open wound.

A potential complication of the tie-over bandage is that the suture loops might cut into the skin if the tie-over strip is tied too tightly. Contamination of the secondary layer of the bandage is possible. However, placing tape or some form of impermeable material over the bandage reduces chances of this complication.

5 Restraint

The use of physical restraining devices to deter an animal from molesting a bandage, cast, or splint should be considered. This is especially needed when the animal will be unsupervised.

Elizabethan collar

Elizabethan collars are an effective way of keeping an animal's teeth and tongue away from a bandage, cast, or splint caudal to the head. They are also effective in keeping paws away from head bandages. Appropriately sized, plastic Elizabethan collars that have loops at the base to accommodate a collar or a length of gauze are the most effective type of collar (fig. 5.1).

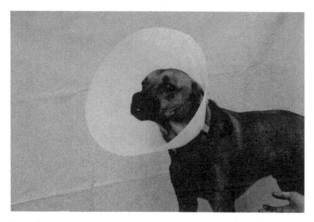

Fig. 5.1. Plastic Elizabethan collar affixed to a dog's leather collar by loops on the Elizabethan collar.

Samll Animal Bandaging, Casting, and Splinting Techniques   Steven F. Swaim, Walter C. Renberg, and Kathy M. Shike
© Steven F. Swaim, Walter C. Renberg, and Kathy M. Shike

Because the collar extends beyond the animal's muzzle, it may be difficult for it to eat and drink from a bowl on the floor. The animal should be observed to see if this is a problem. If it is, several options can be tried. Elevating the bowls may be necessary. Smaller deep bowls that fit inside the collar could be tried. Third, the collar may be removed and then replaced after the animal eats and drinks.

For small dogs, a large plastic bowl can be modified and used similar to the way an Elizabethan collar is used.

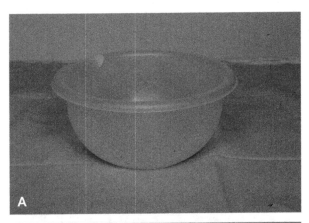

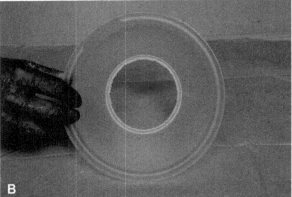

Fig. 5.2.

- A hole through which the animal's head will be placed is cut out of an appropriately sized plastic bowl (figs. 5.2 A and B).

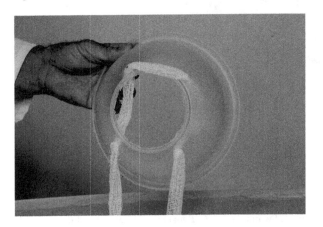

Fig. 5.3.

- Small holes are cut at four equidistant places around the head hole, and a length of gauze is threaded through these holes (fig. 5.3).

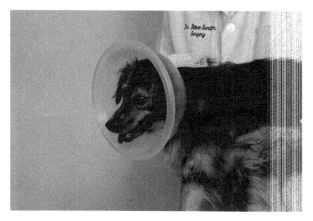

- The dog's head is passed through the large hole and the gauze is tied to secure the bowl in place (fig. 5.4).

Fig. 5.4.

Plastic wrap-around collar

Rigid, plastic wrap-around collars with fasteners (Bite Not Collar, Bite Not Products, San Francisco, CA) can be placed around an animal's neck. They are available in various sizes and extend from just behind the ears to the shoulders. They are equipped with a fabric strap that encircles the thorax just behind the forelimbs. This keeps the collar from coming off over the animal's head (fig. 5.5).

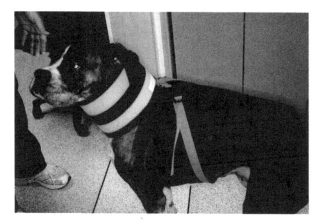

Fig. 5.5. Plastic wrap-around collar with fabric strap around the thorax to keep the collar from coming off over the dog's head.

These collars are effective in keeping an animal from molesting areas caudal to the shoulders. However, they would not be effective in protecting a head bandage. They may not protect the distal limbs from molestation. The collars should be removed daily to check for underlying dermatitis.

Towel collar

A large terry cloth bath towel can be used similar to the way a Bite Not Collar is used.

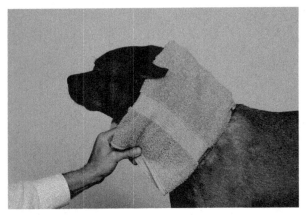

Fig. 5.6.

- A large terry cloth towel is folded such that its width extends from just behind the dog's ears to the shoulders. The folded towel is wrapped around the dog's neck (fig. 5.6).

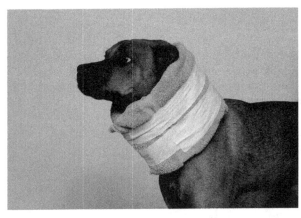

Fig. 5.7.

- Two strips of 2-inch (5.0 cm)-wide adhesive tape are wrapped circumferentially around the towel to hold it in place. Care should be taken not to wrap these too tightly (fig. 5.7).

Muzzles

Muzzles can be used to protect bandages, casts, and splints from teeth and tongues. Cloth and leather muzzles that are used temporarily to protect handlers from animal bites should not be used. These become soaked with saliva, and they are messy and unsanitary. They could also interfere with the dog's breathing or ability to vomit, following sedation, for example. Wire basket-type muzzles should be used.

Wire and plastic basket muzzles are available in various sizes and can be obtained commercially (fig. 5.8). If a dog tends to pull the muzzle off over its nose with its front paws, a strip of 1-inch (2.5 cm)-wide adhesive tape can be folded over on itself lengthwise to provide a means to help prevent this. The strip extends from the portion of the muzzle that is over the nasal area to the strap that goes behind the ears. Thus, it lies up between the eyes. If the muzzle rubs on the side of the face causing a lesion, a larger muzzle should be considered. However, if the lesion is the result of the dog's activity, the area of the muzzle can be padded with a small piece of cotton held in place with some tape.

Side braces

Side braces made from aluminum splint rods can be used to keep a dog away from its hind quarters.

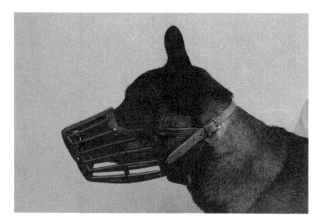

Fig. 5.8. Plastic basket muzzle on a large dog.

- The appropriate size of aluminum splint rod is selected. At its midpoint it is bent into a circle around an object that is approximately the same diameter as the base of the dog's neck on which it will be used (figs. 5.9 A, B, and C).

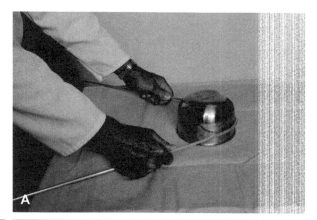

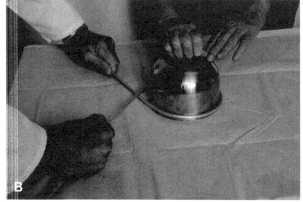

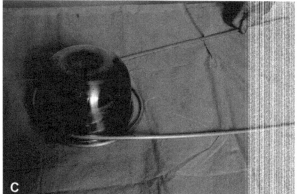

Fig. 5.9.

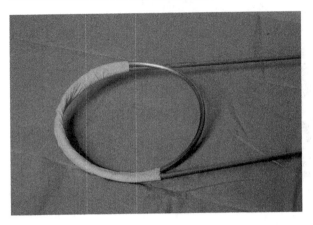

Fig. 5.10.

• Two-inch (5.0 cm)-wide adhesive tape is used to tape the top half of the circle that has two thicknesses of rod (fig. 5.10).

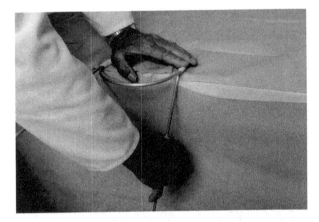

Fig. 5.11.

• The two straight extensions from the circle are bent at a right angle to the circle at the circle's midpoint (fig. 5.11) to provide the basic shape of the brace (fig. 5.12).

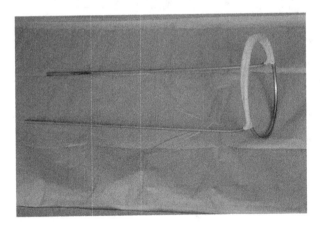

Fig. 5.12.

• The bottom half of the circle is bent back or forward slightly, depending on the dog's anatomy, so this portion of the brace fits the ventral base of the neck better (fig. 5.13).

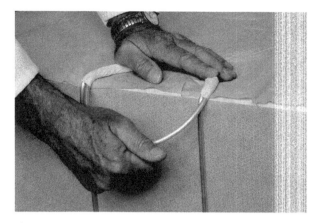

Fig. 5.13.

• Cast padding is wrapped around the bent bottom half of the circle (fig. 5.14).

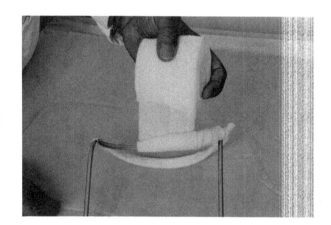

Fig. 5.14.

• Two-inch (5.0 cm)-wide adhesive tape is wrapped over the cast padding (fig. 5.15).

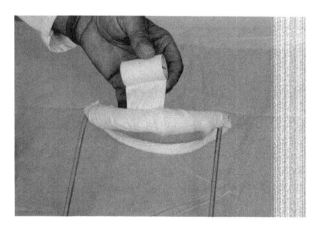

Fig. 5.15.

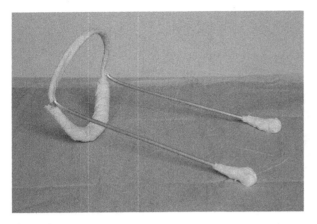

Fig. 5.16.

● The straight extensions are cut with bolt cutters to a length such that they will come to the level of the greater trocanters of the dog. The ends of these extensions are padded with cast padding held in place with adhesive tape (fig. 5.16).

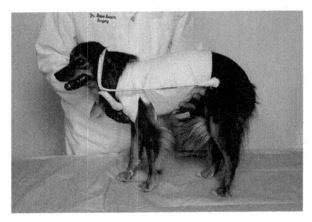

Fig. 5.17.

● A body bandage is applied to the dog (see page 25 chapter 3, Thoracic, Abdominal Bandages). This is followed by placing the splint on the dog such that the circle is at the base of the neck and the side extensions are along the dog's sides. These extensions are held in place by two circumferential wraps of 2-inch (5.0 cm)-wide adhesive tape. One wrap is just behind the forelimbs and the other just in front of the hind limbs (fig. 5.17).

Topical chemical deterrents

Topical chemical deterrents in the form of bitter-tasting materials may be placed on bandages, casts, splints, or around suture lines on intact skin to prevent molestation. These come in various liquid and semiliquid forms and a tape form (fig. 5.18). For best results, a small amount of the material should be placed on or near the dog's nose prior to its use on the bandage, cast, splint, or skin. This allows the animal to lick and smell the substance simultaneously. The substance is then placed on the bandage, cast, splint, or intact skin and the animal will associate the lingering scent with the bitter taste. The authors have had limited success with topical chemical deterrents.

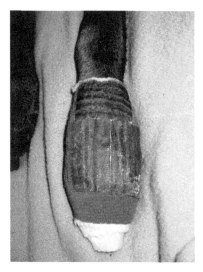

Fig. 5.18. Pepper-impregnated tape on a bandage to deter molestation.

Electronic devices

An additional method to deter animals from licking or removing a bandage, cast, or splint is an electronic product that has a small current. This product (StopLik, Rockway, Inc.) is applied as an adhesive-backed strip that is placed on the outer surface of the bandage. A small battery is included in the strip and a series of exposed metal strips serve as conductors. When the animal licks the bandage, it experiences a small charge. The strips come in a variety of sizes and can be further trimmed to fit (fig. 5.19).

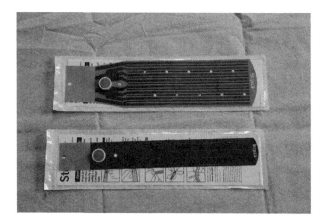

Fig. 5.19. Electronic strips that can be placed on a bandage, cast, or splint to deter molestation.

Suggested Reading

Anderson, Davina. 2009. Management of open wounds. In *BSAVA Manual of Canine and Feline Wound Management and Reconstruction*, 2nd ed., pp. 37–53. Quedgeley, Gloucester, England: British Small Animal Veterinary Association.

Campbell, Bonnie Grambow. 2006. Dressings, bandages, and splints for wound management in dogs and cats. *Veterinary Clinics of North America: Small Animal Practice*. 36(4):759–91. Philadelphia: Saunders/Elsevier.

DeCamp, Charles E. 2003. External coaptation. In *Textbook of Small Animal Surgery*, 3rd ed., pp. 1835–48. Philadelphia: Saunders/Elsevier.

Hedlund, Cheryl S. 2007. Surgery of the integumentary system. In *Small Animal Surgery*, 3rd ed., pp. 159–259. St. Louis: Mosby/Elsevier.

Miller, Craig W. 2003. Bandages and drains. In *Textbook of Small Animal Surgery*, 3rd ed., pp. 244–49. Philadelphia: Saunders/Elsevier.

Pavletic, Michael M. 1999. *Atlas of Small Animal Reconstructive Surgery*, 2nd ed., pp. 107–122. Philadelphia: Saunders.

Scardino, M. Stacie, and Swaim, Steven F. 1997. Bandaging and drainage techniques. In *Current Techniques in Small Animal Surgery*, 4th ed., pp. 27–34. Baltimore: Williams and Wilkins.

Swaim, Steven F., Vaughn, Dana M., Spalding, Patrick R., et al. 1992. Evaluation of the dermal effects of cast padding in coaptation casts on dogs. *American Journal of Veterinary Research* 53(7):1266–72.

Swaim, Steven F., and Henderson, Ralph A. 1997. *Small Animal Wound Management*, 2nd ed., pp. 53–85. Baltimore: Williams and Wilkins.

Swaim, Steven F. 2000. Bandaging and splinting techniques. In *Handbook of Veterinary Procedures and Emergency Treatment*, 7th ed., pp. 549–71. Philadelphia: Saunders.

Swaim, Steven F., Marghitu, Daniel B., Rumph, Paul F., et al. 2003. Effects of bandage configuration on paw pad pressure in dogs: A preliminary study. *Journal of the American Animal Hospital Association*. 39:209–216.

Swaim, Steven F., and Bohling, Mark W. 2005. Bandaging and splinting canine elbow wounds. *NAVC Clinician's Brief*. November: 73–76.

Swaim, Steven, Welch, Janet, and Gillette, Rob. In press. *Small Animal Distal Limb Injuries*. Jackson, WY: Teton NewMedia.

Williams, John, and Moores, Allison. 2009. *BSAVA Manual of Canine and Feline Wound Management and Reconstruction*, 2nd ed., pp. 37–53. Quedgeley, Gloucester, England: British Small Animal Veterinary Association.

Index

Printed in the United States
By Bookmasters